Trauma, Dissociation and Health

This book explores the impact of trauma and dissociation on physical health throughout the lifespan. Important chronic conditions, such as cardiovascular disease and chronic pain, are examined. In addition, trauma in childbearing women is considering, specifically examining the short- and long-term effects of the birth experience itself. Dissociation's effect on long-term health is also described, and how it might manifest in patients in health care settings.

This book was based on a special issue of *Journal of Trauma & Dissociation.*

Kathleen Kendall-Tackett is a health psychologist and an International Board Certified Lactation Consultant. She is a Clinical Associate Professor of Pediatrics at Texas Tech University School of Medicine in Amarillo, Texas, and Acquisitions Editor for Hale Publishing. Dr. Kendall-Tackett is a Fellow of the American Psychological Association in both the Divisions of Health and Trauma Psychology, and is Associate Editor of the journal Psychological Trauma. Dr. Kendall-Tackett is author of more than 240 journal articles, book chapters and other publications, and author or editor of 19 books in the fields of trauma, women's health, depression, and breastfeeding, including *Depression in New Mothers* (2nd Edition, 2010, Taylor & Francis), and *Non-Pharmacologic Treatments for Depression in New Mothers* (2008, Hale Publishing). She is a founding member of the American Psychological Association's Division of Trauma Psychology, and currently serves as Division Secretary.

Bridget Klest is a doctoral student in Clinical Psychology at the University of Oregon, and is completing her predoctoral psychology internship through the University of California San Diego and the San Diego VA Healthcare System. Her research explores the impact of social and interpersonal context on trauma exposure and the development of posttraumatic physical and mental health symptoms. She is currently examining the relations among gender, ethnicity, and access to socio-economic resources as they relate to trauma exposure and posttraumatic symptoms in a Hawaiian cohort.

Trauma, Dissociation and Health

Casual Mechanisms and Multidimensional Pathways

Edited by Kathleen Kendall-Tackett and Bridget Klest

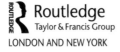

Routledge
Taylor & Francis Group

LONDON AND NEW YORK

First published 2010 by Routledge
2 Park Square, Milton Park, Abingdon, Oxon, OX14 4RN

Simultaneously published in the USA and Canada
by Routledge
711 Third Avenue, New York, NY 10017

Routledge is an imprint of the Taylor & Francis Group, an informa business

First issued in paperback 2013

© 2010 Taylor & Francis

Typeset in Garamond by Value Chain, India

British Library Cataloguing in Publication Data
A catalogue record for this book is available from the British Library

ISBN13: 978-0-415-56528-8 (hbk)
ISBN13: 978-0-415-85175-6 (pbk)

CONTENTS

INTRODUCTION

Causal Mechanisms and Multidirectional Pathways Between Trauma, Dissociation, and Health

KATHLEEN KENDALL-TACKETT, PhD

Department of Pediatrics, Texas Tech University School of Medicine, Amarillo, Texas, USA

BRIDGET KLEST, MA

Department of Psychology, University of Oregon, Eugene, Oregon, USA

Do traumatic events increase the risk of health problems? Over the past decade, researchers in a number of fields—health psychology, medicine, nursing, epidemiology, and public health—have found that they do. In the early stages of this work, researchers worked independently and did not communicate with one another, which limited the application of their findings. For example, researchers in nursing and several fields of medicine—gynecology, gastroenterology, rheumatology—began to notice, quite independently, that patients with pain often had a history of child or domestic abuse (Kendall-Tackett, Marshall & Ness, 2003; Sachs-Ericsson, Cromer, Hernandez, & Kendall-Tackett, this book). Unfortunately, for many years these findings were discounted because the pain syndromes were usually so-called functional conditions (such as irritable bowel syndrome or fibromyalgia), meaning that lab or radiologic findings rarely matched a patient's level of pain or impairment from that pain. Because these findings were not placed in a broader context, symptoms were viewed as idiosyncratic, written off as primarily psychological in origin, and were generally not of interest to health care providers.

In the late 1990s, the first major paper from the Adverse Childhood Experiences Study was to galvanize the issue of trauma and health. The Adverse Childhood Experiences Study included more than 17,000 patients in the Kaiser Permanante Health Maintenance Organization in San Diego, California (Felitti et al., 1998). It was the first large-scale project to conclusively demonstrate that patients who had experienced traumatic events as children had increased risk of developing a number of serious organic diseases, such as cancer, heart disease, diabetes, and chronic obstructive pulmonary disease. The more types of adverse childhood experiences patients experienced, the higher the risk of disease. These findings were too compelling for even the most skeptical health care provider to ignore.

The health of trauma survivors has also been of interest to professionals who work with military populations. Military personnel returning from combat often face a complex combination of physical and psychological injuries. Care providers must understand these relationships as they seek to address the health issues of soldiers returning from Iraq, Afghanistan, and other areas of active deployment (Kinder et al., 2008; Schnurr & Spiro, 1999).

Military research often focuses on the role of posttraumatic stress disorder (PTSD) as a mediator between trauma and health. But PTSD is associated with increased health problems in civilian populations as well. For example, analyzing data from the Canadian Community Health Survey (N = 36,984), researchers found that 1% (n = 478) had a formal diagnosis of PTSD (Sareen et al., 2007). Participants with PTSD had significantly higher levels of hypertension and heart disease; asthma and chronic obstructive pulmonary disease, such as emphysema; chronic pain, including fibromyalgia, arthritis, and migraine; ulcerative colitis and ulcers; and cancer. PTSD was also associated with suicide attempts, poor quality of life, and short- and long-term disability. The authors concluded that these health effects were above and beyond the effects of depression or other mental disorders and were the unique contribution of PTSD.

PTSD following a man-made disaster has shown similar health effects (Dirkzwager, van der Velden, Grievink, & Yzermans, 2007). In this study, 896 survivors of a man-made disaster were surveyed at 3 weeks and 18 months after the disaster. The authors found that PTSD was associated with physician-reported vascular, musculoskeletal, and dermatological problems. PTSD also increased the risk of new vascular problems. These problems appeared even after previous health problems, smoking, and demographic characteristics were controlled.

POSSIBLE PATHWAYS AND CAUSAL MECHANISMS

As we described above, the health effects of trauma are increasingly well documented. But the intriguing question still remains about possible mechanisms for these effects. The presence of health problems in trauma survivors has been well documented. Research on the causal mechanisms connecting traumatic events with health outcomes is more limited. In health psychology research, five possible pathways have been identified, and these are particularly relevant to understanding relationships between trauma and health (Kendall-Tackett, 2003). These pathways are physiological, behavioral, social, emotional, and cognitive. Each pathway alone could lead to poor health. More typically, these pathways co-occur and combine to increase their negative effects. These relationships may also be multidirectional: Trauma influences health along these five pathways, and health can also influence trauma symptoms, with poor health or pain triggering symptoms such as flashbacks, dissociation, anxiety, depression, and intrusive thoughts. We suggest that in a cyclic way, trauma may impact health, further increasing trauma symptoms, which exacerbates health problems.

Pathway Types

The first potential pathway is the physiological changes that can occur in the wake of traumatic events. Indeed, researchers have documented that traumatic events—particularly those that occur in childhood—can alter responsivity of the catecholamine system; the hypothalamic–pituitary–adrenal axis, which regulates the stress hormone cortisol; and the immune system by increasing systemic inflammation and decreasing lymphocyte counts (Kendall-Tackett, 2007; Kibler, this book; Sachs-Ericsson et al., this book).

Some trauma-related changes may also include alterations in sleep, including sleep architecture, which can further exacerbate physiological symptoms such as pain. Sachs-Ericsson and colleagues (this book) discuss chronic pain as another common sequela to trauma. They recognize that the relationship between trauma and pain is not entirely straightforward and likely results from a number of physiological changes caused by trauma exposure, including lowering of the pain threshold, that can increase pain.

Of all of the pathways related to health, behavioral pathways have been studied the most. It has been well documented that trauma survivors often behave in ways that can compromise their health (Davis, Combs-Lane, & Smith, 2004; Kendall-Tackett, 2003; Sachs-Ericsson et al., this book). Behaviors engaged in include substance abuse, smoking, high-risk sexual behaviors, and suicide attempts. These effects may even be intergenerational. Cavanaugh and Classen (this book) examine whether women who have experienced childhood sexual abuse have daughters at increased risk for contracting HIV. They explore this possible relationship by examining whether childhood sexual abuse impacts these women's ability to parent, with special focus on the types of parenting behaviors that decrease the incidence of risky sex among their daughters.

Trauma can also influence survivors by impacting the quality of their social relationships. Without intervention, trauma survivors have higher rates of divorce, more dissatisfaction with adult partners, and greater risk of experiencing revictimization at the hands of a partner or peer. Poor-quality social relationships can impact health in a number of important ways, including by decreasing resilience to stress. In contrast, men and women who have good social support are frequently healthier and live longer than their more isolated counterparts or those in high-strife relationships (Kendall-Tackett, 2003, 2008; Sachs-Ericsson et al., this book). The model that Cavanaugh and Classen present also suggests that a poor mother–daughter relationship may mediate intergenerational transmission of trauma *and* risky health behavior.

Emotional health is another pathway by which trauma can impair physical health. For many years, researchers studying the impact of traumatic events viewed depression, PTSD, and anxiety as primarily out-comes—endpoints in the study. More recently, they have recognized that negative mental states are also mechanisms that can lead to poor health, even increasing the risk of premature mortality (Kendall-Tackett, 2003, 2007; Kibler, this book). For example, in a study of with a large sample of veterans, prior depression (but not PTSD) was associated with increased risk of death 2 years later. This was true even after demographic character-istics, health behaviors, and medical comorbidity were controlled (Kinder et al., 2008).

Another important aspect of trauma and health involves medical settings themselves. Beck (this book) explores how medical settings can actually cause trauma; in this case, when women are giving birth. These effects can last for years, and the impact of these events is rarely acknowledged or treated.

Finally, cognitive pathways can also impact health. What trauma survivors think about themselves and others can dramatically increase their risk of disease. For example, hostility—or framing the world as a dangerous place—is a belief that makes sense in terms of trauma survivors' life experiences. However, hostility has a well-documented negative impact on both cardio-vascular symptoms and the development of diabetes. Similarly, negative beliefs about the self can also lead to poor health (Kendall-Tackett, 2007, in press; Suarez, Lewis, Krishnan, & Young, 2004). For example, shame, a belief common among trauma survivors, can alter the immune system and increase systemic inflammation (Rohleder, Chen, Wolf, & Miller, 2008). These findings are similar to previous studies that have found a link between negative affect states (such as depression and hostility) and inflammation. Prolonged systemic inflammation increases the risk of several chronic diseases, including heart disease and diabetes. The link between negative affect, inflammation, and chronic disease is another possible mechanism by which traumatic events can impact health, even years after the traumatic event (Kendall-Tackett, in press).

Dissociation and Health

Another issue that has not received much attention—but should—is the link between trauma, dissociation, and health. Dissociative symptoms are, of course, associated with trauma, and they can occur because of medical interventions. For example, Beck (this book) describes how a woman's birth experience may be so overwhelming that she dissociates either during labor or postpartum, impacting her ability to function during labor and/or form an attachment with her new baby.

Haven (this book) also discusses the interplay between trauma, dissociation, and health. In her article, Haven describes her work with a client who suffered a brutal attack and then experienced part of his body as "gone." This article chronicles his journey back to where he could feel once again. Haven's description of the therapeutic process for this client makes for interesting reading, and we believe it will help move the dialogue forward on this important issue.

In summary, this book will help researchers and clinicians address both the physical and mental health aspects of traumatic events. By introducing a wide range of perspectives, we hope to offer the reader new ways of looking at the complex, multidirectional relationships between trauma, dissociation, and health. It is our belief that integrating these aspects of trauma survivors' experiences will dramatically improve patient care and more fully address the long-term outcomes of trauma.

REFERENCES

Davis, J. L., Combs-Lane, A. M., & Smith, D. W. (2004). Victimization and health risk behaviors: Implications for prevention programs. In K. A. Kendall-Tackett (Ed.), *Health consequences of abuse in the family: A clinical guide for evidence-based practice* (pp. 179–195). Washington, DC: American Psychological Association.

Dirkzwager, A. J., van der Velden, P. G., Grievink, L., & Yzermans, C. J. (2007). Disaster-related posttraumatic stress disorder and physical health. *Psychosomatic Medicine, 69,* 435–440.

Felitti, V. J., Anda, R. F., Nordenberg, D., Williamson, D. F., Spitz, A. M., Edwards, V., et al. (1998). Relationship of childhood abuse and household dysfunction to many of the leading causes of death in adults: The Adverse Childhood Experiences (ACE) Study. *American Journal of Preventative Medicine, 14,* 245–258.

Kendall-Tackett, K. A. (2003). *Treating the lifetime health effects of childhood victimization.* Kingston, NJ: Civic Research Institute.

Kendall-Tackett, K. A. (2007). Cardiovascular disease and metabolic syndrome as sequelae of violence against women: A psychoneuroimmunology approach. *Trauma, Violence and Abuse, 8,* 117–126.

Kendall-Tackett, K. A. (2008). *Non-pharmacologic treatments for depression in new mothers: Omega-3s, exercise, bright light therapy, social support, psychotherapy and St. John's Wort*. Amarillo, TX: Hale Publishing.

Kendall-Tackett, K. A. (in press). Inflammation, depression and hostility, and risk of disease: The corrosive effects of negative mental states. In K. A. Kendall-Tackett (Ed.), *The psychoneuroimmunology of chronic disease*. Washington, DC: American Psychological Association.

Kendall-Tackett, K. A., Marshall, R., & Ness, K. E. (2003). Chronic pain syndromes and violence against women. *Women and Therapy, 26*, 45–56.

Kinder, L. S., Bradley, K. A., Katon, W. J., Ludman, E., McDonnell, M. B., & Bryson, C. L. (2008). Depression, posttraumatic stress disorder, and mortality. *Psychosomatic Medicine, 70*, 20–26.

Rohleder, N., Chen, E., Wolf, J. M., & Miller, G. E. (2008). The psychobiology of trait shame in young women: Extending the social self-preservation theory. *Health Psychology, 27*, 523–532.

Sareen, J., Cox, B. J., Stein, M. B., Afifi, T. O., Fleet, C., & Asmundson, G. J. (2007). Physical and mental comorbidity, disability, and suicidal behavior associated with posttraumatic stress disorder in a large community sample. *Psychosomatic Medicine, 69*, 242–248.

Schnurr, P. P., & Spiro, A., III. (1999). Combat disorder, posttraumatic stress disorder symptoms and health behaviors as predictors of self-reported physical health in older veterans. *Journal of Nervous and Mental Disease, 187*, 353–359.

Suarez, E. C., Lewis, J. G., Krishnan, R. R., & Young, K. H. (2004). Enhanced expression of cytokines and chemokines by blood monocytes to in vitro lipopolysaccharide stimulation are associated with hostility and severity of depressive symptoms in healthy women. *Psychoneuroendocrinology, 29*, 1119–1128.

Posttraumatic Stress and Cardiovascular Disease Risk

JEFFREY L. KIBLER, PhD

Center for Psychological Studies, Nova Southeastern University, Ft. Lauderdale, Florida, USA

A growing literature indicates that posttraumatic stress is associated with cardiovascular risk and cardiovascular disease (CVD). Research on specific CVD risk factors and their prevalence in posttraumatic stress disorder (PTSD) may improve understanding of CVD development in this population. The primary purpose of the present article is to outline the evidence relating posttraumatic stress to CVD risk, with an emphasis on behavioral factors. The evidence concerning potential elevations in traditional cardiovascular risk factors with behavioral components in PTSD is reviewed. Brief discussions of autonomic nervous system hyperarousal and immune dysfunction as potential mechanisms for CVD risk are also presented. Together, the available evidence suggests that multiple related risk factors and physiological systems may impact health in PTSD. Based on the literature to date, it is suggested that additional studies are needed on the synergistic effects of multiple interacting CVD risk factors and interventions aimed at primary and secondary prevention of cardiovascular risk.

GENERAL OVERVIEW OF THE PROBLEM

A growing literature indicates a relationship between posttraumatic stress disorder (PTSD) diagnosis and cardiovascular problems (Boscarino & Chang, 1999a; Hovens et al., 1998 ; McFarlane, Achison, Rafalowicz, & Papay, 1994; Schnurr, Spiro, & Paris, 2000). Furthermore, one study showed that the relationship of PTSD to physical health was independent of age, depression, or other comorbid anxiety disorders (Zayfert, Dums, Ferguson, & Hegel, 2002). In a study of Vietnam veterans, participants with PTSD were more likely to display an abnormal electrocardiogram (28% vs. 15%) and were more likely to evidence atrioventricular conduction defects and history of myocardial infarction than veterans without PTSD (Boscarino & Chang, 1999a). Cardiovascular disease (CVD) was nearly 2.5 times as common in World War II resistance veterans with PTSD as in a non-veteran, same-age control group (Hovens et al., 1998). Other studies have also identified significantly higher rates of CVD in World War II and Korean veterans with PTSD (Schnurr et al., 2000), as well as in firefighters with PTSD (McFarlane et al., 1994), compared with controls.

Adult cardiovascular problems may be related to childhood trauma for some individuals. Two separate large-scale epidemiological studies in the United States and United Kingdom have demonstrated linear relationships between number of adverse childhood experiences (e.g., abuse or other potentially traumatic event) and cardiovascular risk factors (smoking, obesity, physical inactivity) evidenced as adults (Felitti et al., 1998; Surtees et al., 2003). Data from the U.S. National Comorbidity Survey indicated that among a large representative community sample (n = 5,877), childhood sexual abuse was associated with a more than 3 times greater risk for CVD (Goodwin & Stein, 2004).

Taken together, the literature provides convincing evidence for the association between PTSD and CVD. However, it is not yet clear what the mechanistic pathways are that lead to CVD among individuals with PTSD. There are several potential mechanisms by which PTSD might confer health risks. One hypothesis is that health-related behaviors, which are often related to coping with stress, are affected by posttraumatic stress and directly impact health status. A second hypothesis is that posttraumatic stress has direct deleterious effects on the central nervous system (i.e., altering brain structure or function, or changing the way stimuli are perceived neurologically). A third hypothesis is that immune dysregulation serves as a mediator between stress reactions and health problems among individuals who have experienced traumatic stress. For the purpose of the present article, I focus on the CVD risks that have at least a partial behavioral component (e.g., health risk behaviors and physiological stress reactivity) and the ways in which these reactions may be related to illness. A brief discussion of immune function in PTSD is also included to provide a broader mechanistic context for how behavioral reactions to stress may ultimately be manifested in physical health problems.

CARDIOVASCULAR RISK FACTORS AND POSTTRAUMATIC STRESS

The ways in which people with PTSD cope behaviorally with posttraumatic stress and other stressors in their lives are sometimes unhealthy from a physical standpoint, posing a risk for chronic illnesses such as CVD and HIV. There is some evidence that obesity, high blood pressure (BP), unhealthy lipid levels, cigarette smoking, as well as alcohol abuse may all occur with increased prevalence among individuals with PTSD. From a mechanistic standpoint, some CVD risks have a clearer behavioral coping component (e.g., overeating and smoking), whereas others such as hypertension and hyperlipidemia require dysregulation of physiological processes to progress to a clear CVD risk.

Most studies that have examined cardiovascular risk factors in PTSD have not examined more than one or two risk variables, such as smoking or cholesterol. However, a study of police officers (Violanti et al., 2006) indicated that those with the highest levels of PTSD symptoms were 3 times more likely to exhibit a combination of risk factors (e.g., obesity, high BP, unhealthy lipid profile, elevated glucose levels) that met criteria for metabolic syndrome. Risk factor clustering is of clear conceptual relevance because although CVD risk factors may occur in isolation, clusters are common—for example, obesity and smoking both tend to cluster with elevated BP and unhealthy lipid levels (Perkins, 1985, 1989; Raftopoulos, Bermingham, & Steinbeck, 1999). Prediction of CVD is improved when clusters of multiple risk factors are quantified, as the presence of risk factor clusters may promote the development of atherosclerosis (Berenson et al., 1998).

In a small cross-sectional pilot study recently conducted in our laboratory (Kibler et al., 2007), we assessed five CVD risk variables (i.e., BP, weight, physical inactivity, lipid levels, and smoking) in relation to PTSD status. The pilot study compared CVD risk among relatively young individuals (M age $\pm$ SD = 25 $\pm$ 9 years) with current posttraumatic stress (n = 11) and nonclinical controls (n = 9) with no or minimal PTSD symptoms (and no other mental health conditions). Participants had no prior history of chronic illness, and groups were comparable in terms of gender and race. The PTSD group evidenced significantly more CVD risk factors (M = 1.4) than the control group (M = 0.6). Sample size was not sufficient to test for statistically significant group differences for each risk factor, but effect size calculations indicated a large effect for greater mean weight in the PTSD group (d = .78; respective Ms = 190 lbs vs. 154 lbs), a medium effect for greater diastolic BP in the PTSD group (d = .49; respective Ms = 75.7 mmHg vs. 72.5 mmHg), and a small effect for greater systolic BP in the PTSD group (d = .15; respective

*M*s = 112.2 mmHg vs. 110.0 mmHg). A limitation of our cross-sectional design was that we could not conclude how much of the CVD risk was attributable to PTSD. It is possible that some of the CVD risk factors may have been at elevated levels prior to the individuals experiencing posttraumatic stress and may have been associated with prior stressful life experiences. Although having a control group without posttraumatic stress helps in making some tenuous conclusions, no exclusion for prior trauma exposure was used for the control group.

Obesity and Lipid Levels in PTSD

Although previous studies have indicated comparable mean body weight between PTSD and non-PTSD groups, there is evidence for greater variability in weight and a higher rate of obesity in PTSD among both combat veterans and relatively young women (Lemieux, 1998; Lemieux & Coe, 1995; Shalev, Bleich, & Ursano, 1990). A recent epidemiological study conducted with a nationally representative sample of 12,992 men and women in New Zealand indicated that PTSD was associated with a rate of obesity that was 2.6 times the rate of the general population (Scott, McGee, Wells, & Browne, 2008). This relationship of subsequent obesity to PTSD was twice as strong as that observed for major depression, and it remained significant after controlling for demographic correlates of obesity and PTSD–depression comorbidity.

For those who have been victims of sexual assault or abuse, one hypothesis is that eating serves as a mechanism for coping—several types of traumatic experiences have been associated with binge eating as a way of self-soothing or coping with daily stressors (de Groot & Rodin, 1999; Schwartz & Gay, 1996; Wonderlich et al., 2001). For some individuals who have been abused, binge eating may represent a form of dissociation or a way of focusing attention away from stressful thoughts and negative emotional states (Heatherton & Baumeister, 1991). This theory proposes that trauma survivors engage in a coping strategy of focusing attention on stimuli in the immediate environment in order to avoid more general meaningful or stressful thoughts. This attentional bias facilitates bingeing and unhealthy eating by reducing the normal inhibitions against eating (Heatherton & Baumeister, 1991). Although little information is available to assess whether the nutritional content of foods consumed is different in PTSD, evidence that PTSD may be associated with less nutritional dietary habits can be inferred from studies examining lipid levels. Clinically elevated levels of total cholesterol, low-density lipoprotein cholesterol and triglycerides, and reduced high-density lipoprotein cholesterol have been found to be prominent in Vietnam veterans with PTSD (*M* age = 44 years; Kagan, Leskin, Haas, Wilkins, & Foy, 1999). In a study of Croatian soldiers (*M* age = 34 years), the finding of elevated total cholesterol and triglyceride levels was replicated in mental health patients with PTSD relative to patients without PTSD (Filakovic et al., 1997). Although lipid levels are determined by physiological factors beyond diet, the findings of greater rates of obesity and unhealthy lipid levels in PTSD suggest that overeating, overconsumption of high-fat foods, and/or lack of exercise underlie this contribution to cardiovascular risk.

Another hypothesis concerning body weight in PTSD is that among female sexual abuse survivors, the desire to be overweight serves as a protective mechanism—sexual trauma victims may consider themselves less attractive to other perpetrators by virtue of being overweight (e.g., Weiner & Stephens, 1996). A related phenomenon is the effect of negative self-image on body weight. Women who have been abused commonly have a disrupted sense of self-worth and their own beauty, losing confidence in their ability to be valued and seen as beautiful to others; these beliefs can be manifested in diminished self-care, including overeating and physical inactivity (Robinson, 2000).

Blood Pressure and PTSD

Some individuals with PTSD may be at risk for CVD by virtue of elevated casual BP. Elevated BP is evident in combat veterans with PTSD in both laboratory and 24-hr ambulatory environments (Blanchard, 1990; Buckley & Kaloupek, 2001; McFall, Murburg, Ko, & Veith, 1990; Muraoka, Carlson, & Chemtob, 1998). The study by Muraoka et al. expanded on research that associated PTSD with elevated resting levels of BP by utilizing 24-hr ambulatory monitoring. Among 18 Vietnam veterans, those with PTSD evidenced significantly higher mean diastolic BP readings (80.1 mmHg) across a 24-hr period than veterans without PTSD (71.5 mmHg). Overall, the research examining BP levels in PTSD findings suggests a possible condition of sympathetic nervous system overdrive in PTSD that may be associated with long-term changes in the receptors that regulate BP and risk for hypertension.

In addition to the biological influences, elevated BP is also impacted by behavioral and psychological factors (e.g., Carels, Sherwood, & Blumenthal, 1998; Harrell, 1980). High levels of distress tend to be associated with higher 24-hr BP levels (Kamarck et al., 2005), and interventions to improve stress coping strategies can assist with BP management (e.g., Clifford, Tan, & Gorsuch, 1991; Steptoe, 1988).

The literature on BP in PTSD has lacked a focus on civilians, and few studies have included women. To further explore the issue of hypertension in PTSD by controlling for the potential role of comorbid depression, and to expand this literature beyond the study of combat veterans, we recently conducted an analysis of data from the U.S. National Comorbidity Survey (Kibler, Joshi, & Ma, 2009). The purpose of our study was to examine whether PTSD is significantly associated with hypertension in a community sample, and whether this association is independent of depression. A total of 4,008 National Comorbidity Survey respondents aged 15 to 54 were identified who fit into one of four diagnostic groups: (a) history of PTSD diagnosis (lifetime) and no history of major depression (n = 219), (b) lifetime history of both PTSD and major depression (n = 210), (c) history of major depression (lifetime) and no PTSD (n = 785), and (d) no history of mental illness (n = 2,794). Overall, the rate of hypertension was modest (7.8%) due to the relatively young age of the sample. The rates of hypertension for the group with a history of PTSD and no history of depression (14.5%) and the group with PTSD plus a history of depression (13.9%) were significantly higher than the rates in the no mental illness group (6.5%) and the group with a history of depression and no PTSD (9.7%). These diagnostic group differences in hypertension prevalence were significant when we controlled for a significant positive relationship between age and hypertension rate. The PTSD with no history of depression group did not differ significantly from the PTSD plus history of depression group. We concluded that a history of PTSD is associated with a greater rate of hypertension compared with depression in the absence of PTSD, or no mental illness. The observation that the PTSD with no depression group had a comparable and slightly higher rate of hypertension relative to the PTSD plus depression group suggests that the relationship of PTSD to high BP is independent of comorbid depressive symptoms. Our results also suggest that the findings of higher BP among combat veterans with PTSD may generalize to civilian PTSD samples.

Smoking and PTSD

Smoking is more common among individuals with a history of PTSD, and it is thought to be used as a coping strategy for trauma memories and negative affect (Beckham et al., 1997; Brown, Read, & Kahler, 2003; Shalev et al., 1990; Wyatt, Vargas Carmona, Burns Loeb, & Williams, 2005). In a sample of 98 Israeli combat veterans (M age ± SD = 33 ± 5 years), Shalev and colleagues (1990) observed a smoking rate of 66% among veterans with PTSD compared with 37.5% among veterans without PTSD. Furthermore, smokers with PTSD tend be heavier smokers than controls without PTSD who smoke (Beckham et al., 1997; Shalev et al., 1990). In a sample of 124 help-seeking Vietnam combat veterans with PTSD (M age ± SD = 45 ± 3 years), Beckham et al. (1995) found that smokers had higher levels of PTSD symptoms, suggesting that greater severity of PTSD may contribute to smoking status. The results also suggested that comorbid depressive symptoms were associated with higher levels of smoking among those with higher levels of PTSD (Beckham et al., 1995). Smoking in combination with hypertension and unhealthy lipids increases cardiovascular risk by a factor greater than the sum of their independent risks (Ockene & Houston-Miller, 1997).

Physical Inactivity and PTSD

Physical inactivity is associated with obesity, elevated BP, and a poor lipid profile; conversely, regular physical activity has desirable effects on several important outcomes relevant to cardiovascular risk, such as BP and central body fat (Sallis & Owen, 1999). There is not sufficient evidence to determine if there is a difference in physical activity in PTSD. However, one study showed that high anxiety sensitivity, a common symptom in PTSD, was associated with low exercise motivation among male veterans in treatment for posttraumatic stress (Lyons, McClendon, & Dubbert, 1994). This suggests that heightened concern regarding increases in physical arousal in PTSD may discourage healthy activity levels. This hypothesis is plausible because behavioral avoidance of physiological arousal and startling stimuli represents a hallmark component of PTSD (Meadows & Foa, 1998; Tull & Roemer, 2003). Another study provided evidence that veterans with PTSD are less physically fit than controls based on poorer performance on an ergometric workload test and greater levels of self-reported "effort symptoms," such as shortness of breath and weakness (Shalev et al., 1990).

PHYSIOLOGICAL REACTIVITY AND RECOVERY

In addition to resting or casual measures of physiological parameters such as BP or heart rate, autonomic nervous system (ANS) reactivity to stress has received considerable attention in the PTSD literature. Studies of cardiovascular responses to stress in PTSD have led to the conclusion that there is ANS hyperreactivity in PTSD (e.g., Kosten, Mason, Giller, Ostroff, & Harkness, 1987; Southwick, Yehuda, & Morgan, 1995). Exaggerated cardiovascular reactivity to psychological stress is a proposed mechanism by which negative emotions can confer risk for CVD via chronic overstimulation of the ANS; this "reactivity hypothesis" posits that exaggerated reactivity to mental challenge in the laboratory is representative of increased ANS arousal in response to prolonged psychological stress in the natural environment (Blascovich & Katkin, 1993; Krantz & Manuck, 1984; Obrist, 1981). Heightened cardiovascular reactivity may reflect the negative emotions and altered autonomic control in PTSD during day-to-day environmental stressors (Cohen et al., 1998; Kosten et al., 1987; McFall et al., 1990; Schnurr & Janikowski, 1999; Southwick et al., 1995). Although the mechanisms linking cardiovascular reactivity to CVD risk are not well founded, a tenet of the reactivity hypothesis is that chronic elevations in ANS arousal can confer damage to the walls of blood vessels, lead to changes in receptors that regulate BP (resulting in risk for hypertension), or initiate neuroendocrine responses that increase risk for hypertension and hyperlipidemia (Burker, Fredrikson, Rifai, & Siegel, 1994; Schneiderman et al., 2000; Treiber et al., 2003).

An issue pertinent to the discussion of stress reactivity and PTSD is whether exaggerated ANS responses are specific to trauma-relevant stressors. A large body of research has shown greater cardiovascular reactivity (e.g., heart rate, skin conductance, BP) to trauma-related cues in PTSD (e.g., Orr, Pitman, Lasko, & Herz, 1993; Wolfe et al., 2000). These findings have been interpreted as conditioned learning of hyperarousal of the ANS. However, studies of cardiovascular reactivity in PTSD that have utilized generic, non-trauma-related stress paradigms (e.g., anger recall, mental arithmetic) have revealed mixed results. Some studies have shown that men and women with PTSD exhibit greater reactivity during psychological stress in laboratory settings (Beckham et al., 2002; Goldfinger, Amdur, & Liberzon, 1998; Metzger et al., 1999) and that male veterans with PTSD also have greater ambulatory BP reactivity to distress outside the lab (Beckham et al., 2003; Buckley, Holohan, Greif, Bedard, & Suvak, 2004). Other studies have indicated no differences in reactivity (e.g., McFall et al., 1990; Orr, Meyerhoff, Edwards, & Pitman, 1998; Pitman, Orr, Forgue, de Jong, & Caiborn, 1987; Shalev, Orr, & Pitman, 1993). Among studies yielding no reactivity differences to generic stressors, methodological features have limited interpretation. For example, one study used the period following task instruction and immediately preceding the stress tasks, rather than a pre-instruction rest period, as the pre-stressor baseline (Orr et al., 1998); this method is con-founded by anticipatory reactivity. Studies have also reported using stress reactivity paradigms (Pitman et al., 1987; Shalev et al., 1993) that produced heart rate responses that were very small (less than 3 bpm) and therefore may not have been clinically meaningful experimental manipulations. Taken together, these studies suggest limited preliminary evidence that psychophysiological responses in PTSD are altered in situations that are not trauma related.

In addition to the assessment of cardiovascular reactivity, measurement of cardiovascular recovery from short-term response to stress may prove to be an important index of exaggerated physiological arousal and disease risk (Brosschot & Thayer, 1998; Gregg, James, Matyas, & Thorsteinsson, 1999). Little research to date has examined short-term cardiovascular recovery from stress in PTSD. In one study, higher PTSD symptom levels were asso-ciated with longer heart rate recovery following startle tones (Kibler & Lyons, 2004). In another study, systolic and diastolic BP recovery periods were longer following an anger recall task in veterans with PTSD compared to veterans without PTSD (Beckham et al., 2002). These findings provide preliminary evidence for prolonged cardiovascular responses to stress in PTSD. The recovery period following a stressor may have even more rele-vance than reactivity measures in identifying maladaptive cardiovascular adaptations (Brosschot & Thayer, 1998; Gregg et al., 1999), because slow recovery is thought to reflect extended maintenance of physiological stress reactions.

POTENTIAL IMMUNE MEDIATION OF STRESS AND CVD
RELATIONSHIPS

The available evidence suggests possible cytokine dysregulation in PTSD (e.g., Maes, Lin, Delmeire, Van Gastel, & Kennis, 1999; Spivak et al., 1997). *Cytokines* are protein substances released by cells that serve as intercellular signals to respond to injury and infection. They are an important natural defense mechanism and part of the normal immune response. Proinflammatory cytokines promote inflammation, meaning they attract other immune cells to the site of injury or infection and cause them to become activated to respond. In addition, proinflammatory cytokines are involved in the modulation of anxiety and stress reactions and are released in greater volume when a person is under stress. This increase in the inflammatory response is a potential pathway to multiple disease processes and has been well documented in PTSD (Burges-Watson, Muller, Jones, & Bradley, 1993; Ironson et al., 1997; Maes et al., 1999; Solomon, Segerstrom, & Grohr, 1997; Spivak et al., 1997). In a study that compared 13 patients with PTSD (resulting from either a hotel fire or multiple-collision automobile crash) with 32 healthy controls, levels of the proinflammatory cytokine interleukin-6 were found to be increased in the serum of accident victims with PTSD (Maes et al., 1999). A study that compared 19 veterans with combat-related PTSD with 19 healthy controls revealed higher levels of serum interleukin-1B, another proinflammatory cytokine, in combat veterans with PTSD (Spivak et al., 1997). Levels of interleukin-1B were correlated with duration, but not severity, of PTSD in this study.

Other immune responses have also been found to be altered in PTSD. A study of peripheral blood lymphocytes in patients with PTSD resulting from childhood sexual abuse revealed that 10 women with PTSD had significantly higher levels of lymphocyte activation than 10 age- and gender-matched nonpsychiatric controls, suggesting hyper-elevated immune function (Wilson, van der Kolk, Burbridge, Fisler, & Kradin, 1999). In another study, 10 Vietnam combat veterans with PTSD had significantly higher natural killer (NK) cell activity, and higher numbers of CD4 and CD8 cells, compared to 9 Vietnam combat veteran controls without PTSD (Laudenslager et al., 1998). Boscarino and Chang (1999b) compared the immune profiles of 286 Vietnam veterans with PTSD and 2,179 Vietnam veterans without a psychiatric disorder. In addition to showing that participants with PTSD had significantly higher levels of leukocytes, lymphocytes, and CD4 and CD8 T cell lymphocytes, Boscarino and Chang (1999b) found that participants with PTSD had delayed reactive skin hypersensitivity. This suggests the presence of hypersensitized T cell lymphocytes, which are related to autoimmune diseases such as diabetes and multiple sclerosis (Baker, Mendenhall, Simbarti, Magan, & Steinberg, 1997; Carrithers et al., 1997). In a study that compared women with post-traumatic stress symptoms (related to their child's cancer) and women without posttraumatic stress (with either healthy children or a child with cancer), Glover, Steele, Stuber, and Fahey (2005) found that participants with posttraumatic stress symptoms had significantly higher levels of CD4+ cells, lower levels of CD8+ cells, and blunted natural killer cell activity compared with nonsymptomatic participants. These findings support Boscarino and Chang's (1999b) findings of increased levels of CD4+ cells in male combat veterans with chronic PTSD. However, the low levels of CD8+ conflict with other findings (Boscarino & Chang, 1999b; Laudenslager et al., 1998; Wilson et al., 1999).

The physiological reactivity associated with acute symptomatic PTSD could increase cell-mediated immune function. Cell-mediated immunity is a system that protects against viruses, fungi, and other foreign pathogens. A recent study investigating delayed-type hypersensitivity, a measure of cell-mediated immunity, found significantly increased levels of cell-mediated immunity in women with PTSD related to a childhood history of physical or sexual abuse (Altemus, Cloitre, & Dhabhar, 2003). This finding is consistent with previous work by Burges-Watson and colleagues (1993) indicating increased delayed-type sensitivity in Australian male combat veterans with PTSD, as well as findings of higher plasma levels of proinflammatory cytokines (Maes et al., 1999; Spivak et al., 1997) and increased activation of T lymphocytes (Wilson et al., 1999) in people with PTSD. There is, however, some conflicting evidence, as decreased cell-mediated immunity has been found in Gulf War veterans with PTSD (Schnurr et al., 2000).

SUMMARY AND CONCLUSIONS

The available literature provides compelling evidence that posttraumatic stress is related to CVD risk. A review of the evidence to date suggests that multiple behavioral risk factors, including smoking, high BP, high cholesterol, and obesity, may impact health in PTSD. Although smoking appears to be the most well-established CVD risk factor in PTSD, the available evidence suggests that elevated BP may also be a key factor. Further research is warranted to ascertain whether elevated rates of obesity in PTSD are attributable to physical inactivity, dietary factors, or other behavioral or nonbehavioral factors (e.g., endocrine function). It is also apparent that PTSD is associated with exaggerated physiological reactivity to, and delayed recovery from, stress. To extend the literature to date in the area of PTSD and CVD risk, studies are needed that examine the clustering and synergistic effects of multiple interacting CVD risk factors. Interventions aimed at primary and secondary prevention of cardiovascular risk are also needed.

There is also a growing literature on alterations in immune functioning that are associated with PTSD. Like with the parallel literature on behavioral factors, additional studies to replicate and extend existing findings are needed to draw firm conclusions about the nature of immune dysfunction in PTSD.

Given the evidence concerning stress reactions in PTSD, it is likely that the long-term negative health effects of PTSD are related to a combination of health risk behaviors, such as smoking, poor diet, physical inactivity, and hyperactivity of the ANS. Excess sympathetic nervous system activity may manifest itself through the peripheral immune system, and changes in immune responsivity and cytokine production may well contribute to the deleterious health effects.

REFERENCES

Altemus, M., Cloitre, M., & Dhabhar, F. S. (2003). Enhanced cellular immune response in women with PTSD related to childhood abuse. *American Journal of Psychiatry, 160*, 1705–1707.

Baker, D. G., Mendenhall, C. L., Simbarti, L. A., Magan, L. K., & Steinberg, J. L. (1997). Relationship between posttraumatic stress disorder and self-reported physical symptoms in Persian Gulf War veterans. *Archives of Internal Medicine, 157*, 2076–2078.

Beckham, J. C., Kirby, A. C., Feldman, M. E., Hertzberg, M. A., Moore, S. D., Crawford, A. L., et al. (1997). Prevalence and correlates of heavy smoking in Vietnam veterans with chronic posttraumatic stress disorder. *Addictive Behaviors, 22*, 637–647.

Beckham, J. C., Roodman, A. A., Shipley, R. H., Hertzberg, M. A., Cunha, G. H., Kudler, H. S., et al. (1995). Smoking in Vietnam combat veterans with post-traumatic stress disorder. *Journal of Traumatic Stress, 8*, 461–472.

Beckham, J. C., Taft, C., Vrana, S. R., Feldman, M. E., Barefoot, J. C., Moore, S. D., et al. (2003). Ambulatory monitoring and physical health report in Vietnam veterans with and without PTSD. *Journal of Traumatic Stress, 16*, 329–335.

Beckham, J. C., Vrana, S. R., Barefoot, J. C., Feldman, M. E., Fairbank, J. A., & Moore, S. D. (2002). Magnitude and duration of cardiovascular response to anger in combat veterans with and without chronic posttraumatic stress disorder. *Journal of Consulting and Clinical Psychology, 70*, 228–235.

Berenson, G. S., Srinivasan, S. R., Bao, W., Newman, W. P., III, Tracy, R. E., & Wattigney, W. A. (1998). Association between multiple cardiovascular risk factors and atherosclerosis in children and young adults. *New England Journal of Medicine, 338*, 1650–1656.

Blanchard, E. B. (1990). Elevated basal levels of cardiovascular responses in Vietnam veterans with PTSD: A health problem in the making. *Journal of Anxiety Disorders, 4*, 233–237.

Blascovich, J., & Katkin, E. S. (1993). *Cardiovascular reactivity to psychological stress & disease*. Washington, DC: American Psychological Association.

Boscarino, J. A., & Chang, J. (1999a). Electrocardiogram abnormalities among men with stress-related psychiatric disorders: Implications for coronary heart disease and clinical research. *Annals of Behavioral Medicine, 21*, 227–234.

Boscarino, J. A., & Chang, J. (1999b). Higher abnormal leukocyte and lymphocyte counts 20 years after exposure to extreme stress: Research and clinical implications. *Psychosomatic Medicine, 61,* 378–386.

Brosschot, J. F., & Thayer, J. F. (1998). Anger inhibition, cardiovascular recovery, and vagal function: A model of the link between hostility and cardiovascular disease. *Annals of Behavioral Medicine, 20,* 326–332.

Brown, P. J., Read, J. P., & Kahler, C. W. (2003). Comorbid posttraumatic stress disorder and substance use disorders: Treatment outcomes and the role of coping. In P. Ouimette & P. J. Brown (Eds.), *Trauma and substance abuse: Causes, consequences, and treatment of comorbid disorders* (pp. 171–188). Washington, DC: American Psychological Association.

Buckley, T. C., Holohan, D., Greif, J. L., Bedard, M., & Suvak, M. (2004). Twenty-four-hour ambulatory assessment of heart rate and blood pressure in chronic PTSD and non-PTSD veterans. *Journal of Traumatic Stress, 17,* 163–171.

Buckley, T. C., & Kaloupek, D. G. (2001). A meta-analytic examination of basal cardiovascular activity in posttraumatic stress disorder. *Psychosomatic Medicine, 63,* 585–594.

Burges-Watson, I. P., Muller, H. K., Jones, I. H., & Bradley, A. J. (1993). Cell-mediated immunity in combat veterans with post-traumatic stress disorder. *Medical Journal of Australia, 8,* 55–56.

Burker, E. J., Fredrikson, M., Rifai, N., & Siegel, W. (1994). Serum lipids, neuroendocrine, and cardiovascular responses to stress in men and women with mild hypertension. *Behavioral Medicine, 19*(4), 155–161.

Carels, R. A., Sherwood, A., & Blumenthal, J. A. (1998). Psychosocial influences on blood pressure during daily life. *International Journal of Psychophysiology, 28*(2), 117–129.

Carrithers, M. D. (1997). Immune cell traffic in the brain blundering and migration of autoreactive T lymphocytes. *Neuroscientist, 3,* 207–210.

Clifford, P. A., Tan, S., & Gorsuch, R. L. (1991). Efficacy of a self-directed behavioral health change program: Weight, body composition, cardiovascular fitness, blood pressure, health risk, and psychosocial mediating variables. *Journal of Behavioral Medicine, 14*(3), 303–323.

Cohen, H., Kotler, M., Matar, M. A., Kaplan, Z., Loewenthal, U., Miodownik, H., et al. (1998). Analysis of heart rate variability in posttraumatic stress disorder patients in response to a trauma-related reminder. *Biological Psychiatry, 44,* 1054–1059.

de Groot, J., & Rodin, G. M. (1999). The relationship between eating disorders and childhood trauma. *Psychiatric Annals, 29,* 225–229.

Felitti, V. J., Anda, R. F., Nordenberg, D., Williamson, D. F., Spitz, A. M., Edwards, V., et al. (1998). Relationship of childhood abuse and household dysfunction to many of the leading causes of death in adults: The Adverse Childhood Experiences (ACE) Study. *American Journal of Preventive Medicine, 14,* 245–258.

Filakovic, P., Barkic, J., Kadoic, D., Crncevic-Orlic, Z., Grguric-Radanovic, L., Karner, I., et al. (1997). Biological parameters of posttraumatic stress disorder. *Psychiatria Danubina, 9,* 207–211.

Glover, D. A., Steele, A. C., Stuber, M. L., & Fahey, J. L. (2005). Preliminary evidence for lymphocyte distribution differences at rest and after acute psychological stress in PTSD-symptomatic women. *Brain, Behavior and Immunity, 19,* 243–251.

Goldfinger, D. A., Amdur, R. L., & Liberzon, I. (1998). Psychophysiological responses to the Rorschach in PTSD patients, noncombat and combat controls. *Depression and Anxiety, 8,* 112–120.

Goodwin, R. D., & Stein, M. B. (2004). Association between childhood trauma and physical disorders among adults in the United States. *Psychological Medicine, 34,* 509–520.

Gregg, M. E., James, J. E., Matyas, T. A., & Thorsteinsson, E. B. (1999). Hemodynamic profile of stress-induced anticipation and recovery. *International Journal of Psychophysiology, 34,* 147–162.

Harrell, J. P. (1980). Psychological factors and hypertension: A status report. *Psychological Bulletin, 87,* 482–501.

Heatherton, T. F., & Baumeister, R. F. (1991). Binge eating as escape from self-awareness. *Psychological Bulletin, 110,* 86–108.

Hovens, J. E., Opden Velde, W., Falger, P. R. J., de Groen, J. H. M., Van Duijn, H., & Aarts, P. G. H. (1998). Reported physical health in Resistance veterans from World War II. *Psychological Reports, 82,* 987–996.

Ironson, G., Wynings, C., Schneiderman, N., Baum, A., Rodriquez, M., Greenwood, D., et al. (1997). Posttraumatic stress symptoms, intrusive thoughts, loss, and immune function after Hurricane Andrew. *Psychosomatic Medicine, 59,* 128–141.

Kagan, B. L., Leskin, G., Haas, B., Wilkins, J., & Foy, D. (1999). Elevated lipid levels in Vietnam veterans with chronic posttraumatic stress disorder. *Biological Psychiatry, 45,* 374–377.

Kamarck, T. W., Schwartz, J. E., Shiffman, S., Muldoon, M. F., Sutton-Tyrrell, K., & Janicki, D. L. (2005). Psychosocial stress and cardiovascular risk: What is the role of daily experience? *Journal of Personality, 73,* 1749–1774.

Kibler, J. L., Joshi, K., & Ma, M. (2009). Hypertension in relation to posttraumatic stress disorder and depression in the U.S. National Comorbidity Survey. *Behavioral Medicine, 34,* 125–131.

Kibler, J. L., Joshi, K., Ma, M., Dollar, K. M., Beckham, J. C., Coleman, M., et al. (2007). A pilot study of posttraumatic stress and cardiovascular risk among young adults [Abstract]. *Annals of Behavioral Medicine, 33*(Suppl.), S175.

Kibler, J. L., & Lyons, J. A. (2004). Perceived coping ability mediates the relationship between PTSD symptoms and heart rate recovery in combat veterans. *Journal of Traumatic Stress, 17,* 23–29.

Kosten, T. R., Mason, J. W., Giller, E. L., Ostroff, R. B., & Harkness, L. (1987). Sustained norepinephrine and epinephrine elevation in post-traumatic stress disorder. *Psychoneuroendocrinology, 12,* 13–20.

Krantz, D. S., & Manuck, S. B. (1984). Acute psychophysiological reactivity and risk of cardiovascular disease: A review and methodologic critique. *Psychological Bulletin, 96,* 435–464.

Laudenslager, M. L., Aasal, R., Adler, L., Berger, C. L., Montgomery, P. T., Sandberg, E., et al. (1998). Elevated cytotoxicity in combat veterans with long-term post-traumatic stress disorder: Preliminary observations. *Brain Behavior and Immunity, 12,* 74–79.

Lemieux, A. M. (1998). Abuse-related posttraumatic stress disorder: Challenge to the norepinephrine-to-cortisol hypothesis. *Dissertation Abstracts International*: Section B: The Sciences and Engineering.

Lemieux, A. M., & Coe, C. L. (1995). Abuse-related posttraumatic stress disorder: Evidence for chronic neuroendocrine activation in women. *Psychosomatic Medicine, 57*, 105–115.

Lyons, J. L., McClendon, O., & Dubbert, P. (1994). *Exercise motivation and stages of change in veterans with PTSD*. Abstract presented at the annual meeting of the International Society of Traumatic Stress Studies, November, Chicago, IL.

Maes, M., Lin, A., Delmeire, L., Van Gastel, A., & Kennis, G. (1999). Elevated serum-interleukin 6 (IL-6) and IL-6 receptor concentrations in posttraumatic stress disorder following accidental man-made traumatic events. *Biological Psychiatry, 45*, 833–839.

McFall, M. E., Murburg, M. M., Ko, G. N., & Veith, R. C. (1990). Autonomic responses to stress in Vietnam combat veterans with posttraumatic stress disorder. *Biological Psychiatry, 27*, 1165–1175.

McFarlane, A. C., Achison, M., Rafalowicz, E., & Papay, P. (1994). Physical symptoms in post-traumatic stress disorder. *Journal of Psychosomatic Research, 38*, 715–726.

Meadows, E. A., & Foa, E. B. (1998). Intrusion, arousal, and avoidance: Sexual trauma survivors. In V. M. Follette & J. I. Ruzek (Eds.), *Cognitive-behavioral therapies for trauma* (pp. 100–123). New York: Guilford Press.

Metzger, L. J., Orr, S. P., Berry, N. J., Ahern, C. E., Lasko, N. B., & Pitman, R. K. (1999). Physiologic reactivity to startling tones in women with posttraumatic stress disorder. *Journal of Abnormal Psychology, 108*, 347–352.

Muraoka, M. Y., Carlson, J. G., & Chemtob, C. M. (1998). Twenty-four hour ambulatory blood pressure and heart rate monitoring in combat-related posttraumatic stress disorder. *Journal of Traumatic Stress, 11*, 473–484.

Obrist, P. (1981). *Cardiovascular psychophysiology: A perspective*. New York: Plenum.

Ockene, I. S., & Houston-Miller, N. (1997). Cigarette smoking, cardiovascular disease, and stroke. *Circulation, 96*, 3243–3247.

Orr, S. P., Meyerhoff, J. L., Edwards, J. V., & Pitman, R. K. (1998). Heart rate and blood pressure resting levels and responses to generic stressors in Vietnam veterans with posttraumatic stress disorder. *Journal of Traumatic Stress, 11*, 155–164.

Orr, S. P., Pitman, R. K., Lasko, N. B., & Herz, L. R. (1993). Psychophysiological assessment of posttraumatic stress disorder imagery in World War II and Korean combat veterans. *Journal of Abnormal Psychology, 102*, 152–159.

Perkins, K. A. (1985). The synergistic effect of smoking and serum cholesterol on coronary heart disease. *Health Psychology, 4*, 337–360.

Perkins, K. A. (1989). Interactions among coronary heart disease risk factors. *Annals of Behavioral Medicine, 11*, 3–11.

Pitman, R. K., Orr, S., Forgue, D., de Jong, J., Caiborn, J. (1987). Psychophysiologic assessment of posttraumatic stress disorder imagery in Vietnam combat veterans. *Archives of General Psychiatry, 44*, 970–975.

Raftopoulos, C., Bermingham, M. A., & Steinbeck, K. S. (1999). Coronary heart disease risk factors in male adolescents, with particular reference to smoking and blood lipids. *Journal of Adolescent Health, 25*, 68–74.

Robinson, S. (2000). Body image and body recovery. In A. Y. Shalev & R. Yehuda (Eds.), *International handbook of human response to trauma. The Plenum series on stress and coping* (pp. 163–177). Dordrecht, The Netherlands: Kluwer Academic.

Sallis, J. F., & Owen, N. (1999). *Physical activity & behavioral medicine.* London: Sage.

Schneiderman, N., Gellman, M., Peckerman, A., Hurwitz, B., Saab, P., Llabre, M., et al. (2000). Cardiovascular reactivity as an indicator of risk for future hypertension. In P. M. McCabe, N. Schneiderman, T. Field, & R. A. Wellans (Eds.), *Stress, coping, and cardiovascular disease* (pp. 181–202). Mahwah, NJ: Erlbaum.

Schnurr, P. P., & Janikowski, M. K. (1999). Physical health and post-traumatic stress disorder: Review and synthesis. *Seminars in Clinical Neuropsychiatry, 4,* 295–304.

Schnurr, P. P., Spiro, A., & Paris, A. H. (2000). Physician-diagnosed medical disorders in relation to PTSD symptoms in older male military veterans. *Health Psychology, 19,* 91–97.

Schwartz, M. F., & Gay, P. (1996). Physical and sexual abuse and neglect and eating disorder symptoms. In M. F. Schwartz & L. Cohn (Eds.), *Sexual abuse and eating disorders* (pp. 91–108). New York: Brunner/Mazel.

Scott, K. M., McGee, M. A., Wells, J. E., & Browne, M. A. O. (2008). Obesity and mental disorders in the adult general population. *Journal of Psychosomatic Research, 64,* 97–105.

Shalev, A., Bleich, A., & Ursano, R. J. (1990). Posttraumatic stress disorder: Somatic comorbidity and effort tolerance. *Psychosomatics, 31,* 197–203.

Shalev, A. Y., Orr, S. P., & Pitman, R. K. (1993). Psychophysiological assessment of traumatic imagery in Israeli civilian patients with posttraumatic stress disorder. *American Journal of Psychiatry, 150,* 620–624.

Solomon, G. F., Segerstrom, S. C., & Grohr, P. (1997). Shaking up immunity: Psychological and immunologic changes after a natural disaster. *Psychosomatic Medicine, 59,* 114–127.

Southwick, S. M., Yehuda, R., & Morgan, C. A., III. (1995). Clinical studies of neurotransmitter alterations in post-traumatic stress disorder. In M. J. Friedman, D. S. Carney, & A. Y. Deutch (Eds.), *Neurobiological and clinical consequences of stress: From normal adaptation to PTSD* (pp. 335–349). Philadelphia: Lippincott-Raven.

Spivak, B., Shohat, B., Mester, R., Avraham, S., Gil-Ad, I., Bleich, A., et al. (1997). Elevated levels of serum interleukin-1B in combat-related post-traumatic stress disorder. *Biological Psychiatry, 42,* 345–348.

Steptoe, A. (1988). The processes underlying long-term blood pressure reductions in essential hypertensives following behavioural therapy. In T. Elbert, W. Langosch, A. Steptoe, & D. Vaitl (Eds.), *Behavioural medicine in cardiovascular disorders* (pp. 139–148). Oxford, England: Wiley.

Surtees, P., Wainwright, N., Day, N., Brayne, C., Luben, R., & Khaw, K. (2003). Adverse experience in childhood as a developmental risk factor for altered immune status in adulthood. *International Journal of Behavioral Medicine, 10,* 251–268.

Treiber, F. A., Kamarck, T., Schneiderman, N., Sheffield, D., Kapuku, G., & Taylor, T. (2003). Cardiovascular reactivity and development of preclinical and clinical disease states. *Psychosomatic Medicine, 65,* 46–62.

Tull, M. T., & Roemer, E. (2003). Alternative explanations of emotional numbing of posttraumatic stress disorder: An examination of hyperarousal and experiential avoidance. *Journal of Psychopathology & Behavioral Assessment, 25,* 147–154.

Violanti, J. M., Fekedulegn, D., Hartley, T. A., Andrew, M. E., Charles, L. E., Mnatsakanova, A., et al. (2006). Police trauma and cardiovascular disease: Association between PTSD symptoms and metabolic syndrome. *International Journal of Emergency Mental Health, 8,* 227–238.

Weiner, E. J., & Stephens, L. (1996). Sexual barrier weight: A new approach. In M. F. Schwartz & L. Cohn (Eds.), *Sexual abuse and eating disorders* (pp. 68–77). Philadelphia: Brunner/Mazel.

Wilson, S. N., van der Kolk, B., Burbridge, J., Fisler, R., & Kradin, R. (1999). Phenotype of blood lymphocytes in PTSD suggests chronic immune activation. *Psychosomatics, 40,* 222–225.

Wolfe, J., Chrestman, K. R., Crosby, O. P., Kaloupek, D., Harley, R. M., & Bucsela, M. (2000). Trauma-related psychophysiological reactivity in women exposed to war-zone stress. *Journal of Clinical Psychology, 56,* 1371–1379.

Wonderlich, S. A., Crosby, R. D., Mitchell, J. E., Thompson, K. M., Redlin, J., Demuth, G., et al. (2001). Eating disturbance and sexual trauma in childhood and adulthood. *International Journal of Eating Disorders, 30,* 401–412.

Wyatt, G. E., Vargas Carmona, J., Burns Loeb, T., & Williams, J. K. (2005). HIV-positive black women with histories of childhood sexual abuse: Patterns of substance use and barriers to health care. *Journal of Health Care for the Poor and Underserved, 16*(4), 9–23.

Zayfert, C., Dums, A. R., Ferguson, R. J., & Hegel, M. T. (2002). Health functioning impairments associated with posttraumatic stress disorder, anxiety disorders, and depression. *Journal of Nervous and Mental Disease, 190,* 233–240.

Intergenerational Pathways Linking Childhood Sexual Abuse to HIV Risk Among Women

COURTENAY E. CAVANAUGH, PhD

Department of Psychiatry, Yale University School of Medicine, New Haven, Connecticut, USA

CATHERINE C. CLASSEN, PhD

Department of Psychiatry, University of Toronto, Toronto, Canada

Childhood sexual abuse is prevalent among women, and it has been linked to a number of problems affecting women's health and functioning, including women's parenting practices. Another body of literature has linked specific maternal parenting practices— including mother–daughter sex communication, monitoring/ knowledge about daughters' activities, mother–daughter relationship quality, attitudes toward sex, and modeling of sexual values—to daughters' HIV risk. This article reviews and links these two bodies of literature to indicate how mothers' histories of childhood sexual abuse may compromise their parenting practices, which may in turn impact daughters' HIV risk. We also build upon R. Malow, J. Devieux, and B. A. Lucenko's (2006) model of the associations between childhood sexual abuse and HIV risk to present a model indicating potential intergenerational pathways between child- hood sexual abuse and HIV risk among women. The literature supporting this model and gaps in the literature are described.

This research was supported by Grant T32DA019426 from the National Institute on Drug Abuse.

Childhood sexual abuse (CSA) involving contact (e.g., fondling or sexual intercourse) is experienced by approximately one in three women (Russell, 1983; Wyatt, Loeb, Solis, Carmona, & Romero, 1999) and is linked to a multitude of problems affecting women's health and functioning across the life span (Browne & Finkelhor, 1986; Wyatt, Carmona, Loeb, Ayala, & Chin, 2002). Relatively little research has examined the impact of CSA on mothers' parenting (Maker & Buttenheim, 2000); however, the extant literature suggests that women with histories of CSA are at greater risk for having parenting difficulties (DiLillo & Damashek, 2003). Evidence from the literature on adolescents has also identified specific maternal parenting practices linked with daughters' HIV risk.

The purpose of this article is to review and link these two bodies of literature to indicate potential intergenerational pathways between CSA and HIV risk among women. Furthermore, although there are models of the associations between CSA and HIV risk behaviors (Malow, Devieux, & Lucenko, 2006; Miller, 1999), we are unaware of any models illustrating intergenerational pathways between CSA and HIV risk among women. Therefore, we also build upon Malow and colleagues' (2006) model of the associations between CSA and HIV risk (see Figure 1) and present a model indicating how mothers' histories of CSA may compromise their parenting practices, which in turn may impact daughters' HIV risk (see Figure 2).

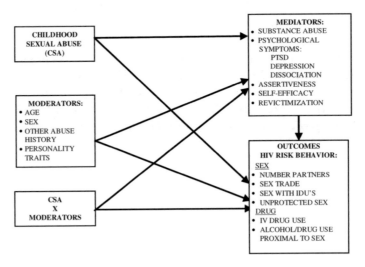

FIGURE 1 Childhood sexual abuse and HIV risk: A proposed model of the association. PTSD = posttraumatic stress disorder; IDU = injection drug use; IV = intravenous. From "History of childhood sexual abuse as a risk factor for HIV risk behavior," by Malow, R., Devieux, J., & Lucenko, B. A., 2006, *Journal of Psychological Trauma, 5*(3), 13–32. Reprinted by permission of Taylor & Francis, http://www.informaworld.com.

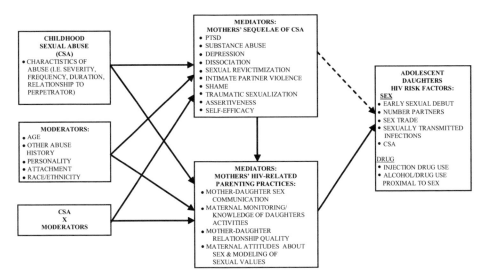

FIGURE 2 Childhood sexual abuse and HIV risk: Intergenerational pathways among women. Solid lines indicate that, in general, all variables in one box are posited to impact the variables in the other box. Dashed lines indicate that only some variables are posited to impact variables in the adjoining box. PTSD = posttraumatic stress disorder; IV = intravenous.

CSA AND ASSOCIATED SEQUELAE

CSA has been associated with subsequent psychological problems and victimization. Common mental health problems associated with CSA include posttraumatic stress disorder (PTSD; Rodriguez, Vande Kemp, & Foy, 1998), substance use problems (Simpson & Miller, 2002), and depression (Weiss, Longhurst, & Mazure, 1999). In a nationally representative study, women's CSA was significantly associated with the subsequent onset of 14 of 17 mood, anxiety, and substance use disorders after controlling for other childhood adversities (Molnar, Buka, & Kessler, 2001). Furthermore, the risk for psychiatric disorders seems to increase with CSA severity. Worse sequelae have been associated with childhood attempted or completed rape than childhood molestation followed by noncontact abuse (e.g., indecent exposure; Fergusson, Horwood, & Lynskey, 1996; Molnar et al., 2001). Dissociation (Briere & Runtz, 1988), sexual revictimization (Classen, Palesh, & Aggarwal, 2005), and intimate partner violence (Feerick, Haugaard, & Hien, 2002) are also more common among women with histories of CSA than among nonabused women. Many victims of CSA also report feelings of shame that may persist over time (Browne & Finkelhor, 1986; Feiring & Taska, 2005).

CSA also undermines women's sexual health, functioning, and satisfaction (Browne & Finkelhor, 1986; Loeb et al., 2002). Finkelhor and Browne

(1985) described how CSA may inappropriately shape sexuality, leading to traumatic sexualization by teaching a child not only misconceptions about sexual behavior and sexual morality but (a) to use sexual behavior for manipulating others and (b) to link frightening memories with sexual activity. There is empirical evidence linking CSA with several measures of women's sexuality, including more liberal sexual attitudes (Meston, Heiman, & Trapnell, 1999). Women with histories of CSA have also been found to report more negative sexual affect, including anger and fear, during sex acts and to perceive themselves as being less romantic/passionate (Meston, Rellini, & Heiman, 2006). Evidence suggests that the relationship between CSA and higher levels of negative sexual affect is mediated by CSA survivors having lower levels of romantic/passionate sexual self-schemas (Meston et al., 2006). Survivors of CSA have also been found to have less sexual assertiveness (Johnsen & Harlow, 1996) and condom self-efficacy (Brown, Lourie, Zlotnick, & Cohn, 2000) compared to peers without such histories. CSA is also linked with risky HIV sex behaviors among women, including unprotected sexual intercourse, sex with multiple partners, trading sex, and adult sexual revictimization (Arriola, Louden, Doldren, & Fortenberry, 2005; Senn, Carey, & Vanable, 2008), with greater HIV risk associated with more severe CSA histories (Senn, Carey, Vanable, Coury-Doniger, & Urban, 2007).

CSA AND PARENTING PRACTICES

Fewer studies have examined the adverse impact of CSA on parenting (Maker & Buttenheim, 2000; Ruscio, 2001). Nevertheless, the extant literature suggests that CSA is a risk factor for some parenting problems among women, including difficulty establishing appropriate hierarchical boundaries, permissive parenting, and the use of physical discipline (DiLillo, 2001; DiLillo & Damashek, 2003). Cohen (1995) compared mothers with histories of CSA to those without on seven parenting skills and found that mothers with histories of CSA had lower mean scores on each of the parenting skills, including communication, limit setting, and role image. In another study, CSA was associated with less maternal confidence after adjusting for physical and emotional abuse in childhood (Roberts, O'Connor, Dunn, & Golding, 2004). After controlling for childhood physical abuse, neglect, and negative family relationships, Banyard (1997) found that CSA among mothers was associated with more use of physical violence as a strategy for dealing with parent–child conflict and with mothers wanting to change more about themselves as parents. Mothers with histories of CSA have also been found to be more emotionally dependent upon their child than nonabused mothers (Burkett, 1991), particularly if they are dissatisfied with their relationship with their partner (Alexander, Teti, & Anderson, 2000). Furthermore, when 40 women with histories of childhood or adolescent incest were interviewed about their experience as a parent, Armsworth and Stronck (1999) reported that

> the most frequent response was "detached or numb.' Thirty percent stated that they felt 'handicapped' by a lack of skills or models for parenting, and 25% stated that they felt helpless or overwhelmed by parenting for similar reasons. Nearly a third described their behavior as being 'overcontrolling and over-protective,' and an equal number described the situations they created as being impulsive, abusive, or reenactments of their own past. (p. 308)

Mothers who are survivors have also reported difficulties with trusting others, not knowing about what constitutes normal development, and keeping boundaries (Cross, 2001). Despite the accumulating literature suggesting that women with histories of CSA have greater difficulty parenting (DiLillo & Damashek, 2003), we are aware of only one parenting intervention for mothers with histories of CSA (Hiebert-Murphy & Richert, 2000).

PARENTING PRACTICES ASSOCIATED WITH ADOLESCENT HIV RISK

Another body of literature has linked specific parenting practices—including parent–adolescent sex communication, parental monitoring/knowledge, parent–adolescent relationship quality, and parental attitudes toward sex and modeling of sexual values (Crosby & Miller, 2002; Kotchick, Shaffer, & Forehand, 2001)—to adolescents' HIV risk. We refer to such parenting practices as *HIV-related parenting practices*. Although this literature has largely focused on general parenting practices and adolescent risk behavior, we focus on the relationships between maternal HIV-related parenting practices and adolescent daughters' HIV risk for several reasons. There is evidence suggesting that mothers in particular may influence adolescent girls' sexual health (Crosby & Miller, 2002). The context of sexual development, including HIV risk, is also different for girls than boys. Girls are four times more likely than boys to experience CSA involving vaginal, oral, or anal intercourse (Fergusson, Lynskey, & Horwood, 1996). This directly increases adolescent girls' HIV risk exposure. Furthermore, gender identity and gender role socialization shape the sexual attitudes and behaviors of girls differently than those of boys (Amaro, Navarro, Conron, & Raj, 2002). These variables interact with other cultural variables, including those that limit women's economic power and control of resources, to affect girls' and women's HIV risk behavior (Logan, Cole, & Leukefeld, 2002; Wingood & DiClemente, 2000). As such, gender-specific examinations of HIV risk are warranted. A related literature review follows.

Mother–Daughter Sex Communication

Several aspects of mother–daughter sex communication, including the process, number of topics covered, and the frequency of communication about birth control or sexual values, have been linked to adolescent girls' sexual risk taking (Dutra, Miller, & Forehand, 1999; Henrich, Brookmeyer, Shrier, & Shahar, 2006; Hutchinson, Jemmott, Jemmott, Braverman, & Fong, 2003; Luster & Small, 1994) and history of sexual intercourse (Usher-Seriki, Smith Bynum, & Callands, 2008). Black and Hispanic adolescent girls who reported (a) having a more open and receptive process of sex communication with mothers or (b) covering more content of sexual communication with their mothers were less likely to engage in sexual risk taking (Dutra et al., 1999). The number of sexually related topics (e.g., sexual intercourse, birth control, AIDS, sexually transmitted diseases, condoms) about which urban African American and Latina adolescent girls talked to their mothers was also associated with fewer episodes of sexual intercourse and unprotected intercourse at a 3-month follow-up (Hutchinson et al., 2003). There was also evidence suggesting that mother–daughter sex communication predicted fewer sexual partners, but this finding did not reach statistical significance.

Luster and Small (1994) found that predominantly White, 13- to 19-year-old adolescent girls who reported less frequent communication with their mothers about birth control had higher sexual risk, such as having more than one sexual partner and rarely or never using contraception. Other studies suggest that mother–daughter communication about sex may interact with other parenting variables, including parent–child relationship quality, to influence girls' HIV risk. In a national longitudinal study, less extensive mother–daughter sex communication in the context of lower parent connectedness was associated with adolescent girls being more likely to engage in sexual risk behavior a year later, including not having used a condom in the past year, drinking or using drugs during their most recent sexual encounter, exchanging sex, and having ever had anal sex (Henrich et al., 2006). Although mothers' perceptions of more frequent conversations about general sex topics were linked to increased odds of African American adolescent girls having engaged in sexual intercourse, mothers' perceptions of more frequent conversations about sexual values were associated with decreased odds of girls engaging in sexual intercourse in the same population (Usher-Seriki et al., 2008). These findings suggest that aspects of sex communication may be differentially related to adolescent girls' sexual behavior.

Parental Monitoring/Knowledge

Parental monitoring/knowledge has also been linked to girls' HIV risk behavior. *Parental monitoring* has been described as parents' "attention to and tracking of the child's whereabouts, activities, and adaptations" (Dishion & McMahon, 1998, p. 61). Some argue that it is really knowledge that parents have about what their children are doing outside the home, and that this knowledge is acquired from parents' own efforts to learn about their children's activities and from what children tell parents about their activities (Stattin & Kerr, 2000). We do not enter the debate here but rather provide a brief summary of the literature in the area of parental monitoring/knowledge as associated with adolescent girls' risky sex behavior.

Most studies have examined parental monitoring as a general concept in relation to adolescent girls' HIV risk with little attention to the potential unique effects of maternal versus paternal monitoring. Nevertheless, a number of studies have shown relationships between adolescent girls' reports of what their parents inquire about and know regarding how they spend their time and their sexual risk (Crosby, DiClemente, Wingood, Lang, & Harrington, 2003; DiClemente et al., 2001; Luster & Small, 1994; Rodgers, 1999). Evidence from one study showed that parental monitoring related to girls' HIV risk was done primarily by mothers (DiClemente et al., 2001). Luster and Small (1994) and Rodgers (1999) found that primarily White teenage girls who perceived their parents knew less about their whereabouts and showed less interest in how and with whom they spent their free time had increased odds of being in a high sexual risk group, whereas those who reported more parental monitoring/knowledge were more likely to be in the low sexual risk group. In a prospective study, African American female adolescents who reported infrequent parental monitoring at baseline were found to be more likely to test positive for a sexually transmitted infection 18 months later compared to peers who reported frequent parental monitoring (Crosby et al., 2003). In another study, sexually active Black adolescent girls who reported that their parents knew less about where and with whom they spent their time away from home were more likely to test positive for a sexually transmitted disease, to report not having used a condom during their most recent sexual intercourse, and to report not having used any kind of contraception during their past five intercourse occasions compared to their peers who reported that their parents knew more about their activities (DiClemente et al., 2001). Adolescent girls reporting more parental knowledge about their activities were also marginally more likely to report having had multiple sex partners in the past six months or a non-monogamous sexual partner. This study, which is unique for noting that the primary provider of parental monitoring was mothers, provides evidence linking maternal monitoring/knowledge to adolescent girls' sexual risk taking.

Mother–Daughter Relationship Quality

Adolescent girls' parent–child (Henrich et al., 2006) and mother–daughter (Dittus & Jaccard, 2000; Usher-Seriki et al., 2008) relationship quality have been linked to their sexual risk and history of sexual intercourse. As previously mentioned, adolescent girls' reports of less parent connectedness (e.g., how close they felt to their mother/father or how warm and loving their mother/father was most of the time) in the context of less extensive mother–daughter sex communication was associated with increased odds of girls' subsequent sexual risk behavior a year later (Henrich et al., 2006). The degree to which adolescents reported being satisfied with their maternal relationship has also been associated with a lower odds of engaging in sex or becoming pregnant and higher odds of using birth control approximately one year later (Dittus & Jaccard, 2000). More positive mother–daughter relationship quality, as measured by African American adolescent girls' responses to five questions (including whether their mothers were warm and loving most of the time, and their overall satisfaction with their relationship with their mother), has also been associated with a lower likelihood of girls having engaged in sexual intercourse (Usher-Seriki et al., 2008).

Maternal Attitudes Toward Sex and Modeling of Sexual Values

There is also evidence linking maternal attitudes toward sex and modeling of sexual values to adolescent girls' sexual behavior (Crosby & Miller, 2002; Dittus & Jaccard, 2000; Kotchick, Dorsey, Miller, & Forehand, 1999; Kotchick et al., 2001; Usher-Seriki et al., 2008; Whitbeck, Simons, & Kao, 1994). Whitbeck and colleagues noted that higher rates of sexual activity among adolescents living in single-parent households may be explained by the fact that adolescents may be more aware of their mothers' dating relationships and sexuality than those in two-parent households. These researchers studied the relationships between mothers' dating, adolescents' and mothers' sexual attitudes, and adolescents' sexual activity. A daughter's sexual activity was associated with (a) how soon after divorce her mother began dating; (b) her mother's sexual permissiveness (e.g., how wrong the mother thought it was for her child to have sexual intercourse or to have a child); and (c) the daughter's own sexual permissiveness, as indicated by her ratings of the contexts for which sexual activity was acceptable (Whitbeck et al., 1994). Daughters' ratings of the contexts for which sexual activity was acceptable were in turn associated with mothers' sexual permissiveness and mothers' dating (e.g., number of dating partners, frequency of dating, and how soon after divorce mother began dating).

Both mothers' actual attitudes about sex and adolescents' perceptions of maternal attitudes about sex have been linked to girls' sexual behavior (Dittus & Jaccard, 2000). Maternal disapproval and adolescents' perceptions of their mothers' disapproval of sex were both associated with a lower likelihood adolescents would have sexual intercourse a year later; however, only adolescents' perceptions of their mothers' disproval were associated with a lower likelihood of adolescent girls becoming pregnant one year later. It is interesting that neither mothers' disapproval nor girls' perceptions of their mothers' disapproval was linked to adolescents having used birth control during their most recent sexual episode. Nevertheless, these findings suggest that the both maternal attitudes about sex and adolescents' perceptions of them may be important variables to consider in relation to girls' HIV risk behaviors.

Additionally, in a sample of Black and Hispanic single-mother families, mothers' sexual risk taking (e.g., number of men she had sex with and times she had used a condom in the past year) was positively associated with adolescent sexual risk taking, though the relationship disappeared when mother–adolescent sex communication and maternal attitudes about adolescent sexuality were controlled (Kotchick et al., 1999). Furthermore, adolescent girls who perceived greater maternal approval of premarital sex were more likely to have had sexual intercourse compared to adolescent girls who perceived less maternal approval of premarital sex (Usher-Seriki et al., 2008). This body of literature suggests that mothers' (a) real and perceived sexual attitudes and modeling of sexual values, (b) communication with daughters about sex, (c) parental monitoring/knowledge about their daughters' activities, and (d) relationship quality with daughters are important maternal parenting behaviors linked to girls' sexual behavior and risk. It is therefore essential to identify mothers who may have particular difficulty in these areas in order to inform prevention and intervention efforts to strengthen maternal HIV-related parenting practices and reduce HIV risk in the next generation of girls.

DO MOTHERS WITH HISTORIES OF CSA HAVE POORER HIV-RELATED PARENTING PRACTICES?

Although the evidence reviewed above suggests that women with histories of CSA may have greater difficulties parenting than nonabused women and that specific maternal parenting practices may be linked to a daughter's HIV risk, we are unaware of studies examining whether a mother's history of CSA affects parenting practices that are known to be linked to a daughter's HIV risk. Nevertheless, we link these two bodies of literature below to indicate pathways by which mothers' histories of CSA may be linked to daughters' HIV risk. We build upon Malow and colleagues' (2006) model of the associations between CSA and HIV risk and propose a model indicating potential intergenerational pathways linking CSA and HIV risk among women (see Figure 2).

CSA and its sequelae may affect mothers' communication with their daughters about sex, monitoring of their daughters' activities, relationships with their daughters, and attitudes about sex and modeling of sexual values. Some examples of such difficulties have been evident in our clinical and research experience with adult female survivors of CSA. Women with histories of CSA may have a particularly difficult time talking to their daughters about sex. For many women, talking to their daughters about sex may result in their daughters asking them about their own sexual experiences. Mothers with histories of CSA who anticipate such questions may avoid talking to their daughters about sex in order to avoid being confronted with their own traumatic sexual experiences. Furthermore, given evidence that mothers' knowledge, skills, comfort, and confidence are positively associated with discussions with their children about sex (Miller et al., in press), and given the potential for mothers with histories of CSA to feel uncomfortable and unconfident talking with their children about sex, there may be a greater likelihood for mothers with such histories to avoid conversations about sex with their daughters. Additionally, evidence suggesting that female survivors of CSA have more liberal sexual attitudes (Meston et al., 1999) suggests that these mothers might communicate more liberal attitudes about sex to their daughters than mothers without such histories.

Many mothers with histories of CSA lack trust about leaving their daughters with others and have reported overly monitoring their daughters in order to protect them from sexual assault. Mothers' concern and efforts to protect their children may also impact their daughters and their relationships with them. For example, one female survivor reported repeatedly examining her daughter's underwear and body for signs of sexual assault, and other women have described not wanting female children in order to avoid worrying about their daughters' safety. Additionally, higher rates of risky sex practices, including sex trade and multiple partners, among CSA survivors (Senn et al., 2008) may be visible to the daughters of these women even if the mothers do not suspect their daughters are aware of such behaviors. For example, some children may know their mothers engage in sex work, others may be aware that their mothers have multiple sexual partners, and some may learn about their mothers' sexuality through overhearing their mothers' conversations with others or through direct conversations. Evidence suggesting that some women with histories of CSA may engage in role reversal (Alexander et al., 2000; Burkett, 1991) with their children suggests that potentially inappropriate conversations may occur between mothers and daughters. Daughters' knowledge of such behaviors may impact their perceptions about their mothers' sexual attitudes and, in turn, the daughters' own sexual behavior, including HIV risk.

RELATIONSHIPS BETWEEN SEQUELAE OF MOTHERS' CSA AND HIV-RELATED PARENTING PRACTICES

The sequelae of CSA may also be related to mothers' HIV-related parenting practices, although there is a paucity of research examining these relationships. For example, the more posttraumatic symptoms a mother experiences in response to her sexual victimization, the greater difficulty she may have talking to her child about sex because doing so may act as a trigger for the mother. Furthermore, some of the sequelae associated with CSA, particularly those that compromise mothers' mental health and functioning (such as substance abuse, depression, and PTSD), may undermine women's abilities to monitor their children effectively. There is evidence linking dissociation to lack of monitoring and supervision (Collin-Vezina, Cyr, Pauze, & McDuff, 2005).

Furthermore, PTSD, depression, and intimate partner violence have been linked to poorer parenting satisfaction and perceptions (Samper, Taft, King, & King, 2004; Schuetze & Eiden, 2005), mothers' distorted mental representations of their children and their relationships with their children (Schechter et al., 2005), and children's impaired self- and other mental representations (Schechter et al., 2007), all of which are likely to compromise parent–child relationship quality. PTSD, drug use, and intimate partner violence have also been linked to women's sexual risk taking and sexual revictimization (Coker, 2007; El-Bassel et al., 1998; Risser, Hetzel-Riggin, Thomsen, & McCanne, 2006; Senn, Carey, Vanable, Coury-Doniger, & Urban, 2006), which may thereby affect mothers' modeling of sexual values. Finally, evidence demonstrating that depression and intimate partner violence (Schuetze & Eiden, 2005) mediate the relationships between CSA and parenting practices suggests that these and other sequelae of abuse may also mediate the relationships between mothers' histories of CSA and HIV-related parenting practices.

RELATIONSHIPS BETWEEN SEQUELAE OF MOTHERS' CSA AND ADOLESCENT HIV RISK

Some sequelae of CSA among mothers may also have a direct relationship with adolescent daughters' risky sex and sexual victimization, placing the latter at risk for HIV. For example, adolescents who witnessed family violence were 3.6 times more likely than adolescents who had not witnessed family violence to have sex without condoms (Voisin, 2005). Drug use among mothers with a history of CSA (McCloskey & Bailey, 2000) and maternal psychiatric illness have also been identified as risk factors for CSA among children (Sidebotham, Golding, & the Alspac Study Team, 2001), which may increase adolescent girls' HIV risk exposure. These findings suggest that sequelae associated with mothers' histories of CSA—including maternal substance abuse, psychiatric illness, and intimate partner violence—may directly influence adolescent girls' CSA exposure and sexual risk taking.

MODERATORS

Finally, other factors may moderate the proposed relationships between CSA and the variables captured in our model as mediators. Varying rates of intimate partner violence and substance abuse by age (Substance Abuse and Mental Health Services Administration, 2006; U.S. Department of Justice, 2007) suggest that some of the relationships with those variables proposed in this model may be moderated by age. CSA is correlated with other types of abuse, including childhood physical abuse, emotional abuse, and neglect (Dong, Anda, Dube, Giles, & Felitti, 2003), and those other forms of abuse may also influence the relationships between CSA and other variables in the model. Childhood abuse is linked with personality disorders (Battle et al., 2004; Fossati, Madeddu, & Maffei, 1999), which in turn are associated with other co-occurring psychological disorders such as those identified as sequelae of CSA (Oldham et al., 1995). Maternal personality has also been linked with parenting behaviors (Desjardins, Zelenski, & Coplan, 2008; Smith et al., 2007), and there is evidence that personality characteristics may be linked to HIV risk behaviors such as parental modeling of sexual values (Trobst, Herbst, Masters, & Costa, 2002). Therefore, personality may moderate relationships in the model. Furthermore, the development of psychopathology in response to traumatic events such as CSA is influenced by attachment relationships (Charuvastra & Cloitre, 2008; Riggs et al., 2007). Finally, given findings that race/ethnicity moderated the relationships between domestic violence victimization and substance abuse (Sullivan, Cavanaugh, Ufner, Swan, & Snow, in press) and racial/ethnic differences in parental communication about sex (Hutchinson, 2002; Meneses, Orrell-Valente, Guendelman, Oman, & Irwin, 2006), parental monitoring (Crosby et al., 2006), and substance use disorders (Substance Abuse and Mental Health Services Administration, 2006), race/ethnicity is also indicated as a potential moderator of the relationships modeled in Figure 2.

DISCUSSION

We have provided a brief review of the literature summarizing (a) how CSA affects women's functioning, including parenting practices; and (b) how specific maternal parenting practices are associated with daughters' risk of HIV infection. We have linked these two bodies of literature to indicate how mothers' histories of CSA may be associated with daughters' HIV risk and have presented a model indicating potential intergenerational pathways linking mothers' CSA to daughters' HIV risk. This model illustrates how a mother's history of CSA along with other characteristics may either directly affect or moderate specific outcomes, such as (a) maternal substance abuse, PTSD, and intimate partner violence; and (b) maternal HIV-related parenting practices (e.g., mother–daughter sex communication, monitoring/knowledge of daughters activities, mother–daughter relationship quality, and maternal attitudes about sex and modeling of sexual values), which in turn impact daughters' HIV risk. As reviewed and illustrated in the model, problems associated with CSA among mothers may be related to daughters' HIV risk indirectly (through affecting mothers' HIV-related parenting practices) and directly (through relationships between some of the sequelae of CSA among mothers—including intimate partner violence and substance abuse—having direct relationships with daughters' HIV risk).

This review and the model of relationships depicted are not intended to be an exhaustive summary of all of the relationships linking mothers' histories of CSA with daughters' HIV risk or affecting adolescent girls' HIV risk. Our goal here was to review and link two bodies of literature in order to identify some of the potential pathways linking CSA to HIV risk among women. There are, of course, other variables that influence girls' HIV risk (Donenberg & Pao, 2005), including friends' behaviors and attitudes as well as other pathways that may link maternal CSA to girls' HIV risk, that warrant consideration in relation to the variables discussed. Additionally, although many of the relationships in this model may also apply to fathers and adolescent boys, we focused this review specifically on the intergenerational transmission of HIV risk among women for the reasons already stated, including evidence suggesting that mothers in particular influence their daughters' sexual health (Crosby & Miller, 2002; Whitbeck et al., 1994). Intergenerational models linking CSA to HIV risk among men are also needed. Finally, although the literature reviewed focused on adolescent girls' risky sex practices or victimization (including unprotected sex, the number of sexual partners, and CSA), we included injection drug use and early sexual debut in our model as adolescent daughters' HIV risk factors, as we suspect that these HIV risk behaviors among girls may also be related to the maternal mental health functioning and HIV-related parenting practices that we suggest may be compromised among mothers with histories of CSA.

FUTURE DIRECTIONS

There are calls for more research examining the associations between CSA and subsequent parenting (DiLillo & Damashek, 2003)—such as the relationship between CSA severity and dysfunctional parenting and the impact of sequelae of CSA on parenting difficulties—in order to inform appropriate interventions (Ruscio, 2001). Given the evidence linking mothers' communication with daughters about sex, their monitoring and knowledge of daughters' activities, mother–daughter relationship quality, and their attitudes about sex and modeling of sexual values with daughters' HIV risk behaviors (Crosby & Miller, 2002; Kotchick et al., 2001), research on these parenting behaviors among mothers with histories of CSA may elucidate parenting difficulties and inform interventions to strengthen parenting skills in this population of women and to prevent HIV risk in their daughters. Specifically, future research should address the following questions: Do mothers with histories of CSA, particularly those who were severely traumatized, differ from women without histories of CSA in (a) how they talk to their daughters about sex, (b) their parental monitoring/knowledge of their daughters' activities, (c) their mother–daughter relationship quality, or (d) their attitudes about sex and modeling of sexual values? If so, do the sequelae associated with CSA mediate the relationships between mothers' histories of CSA and mothers' HIV-related parenting practices? Studies exploring how mothers with histories of CSA deal with their daughters' sexuality in general may also clarify other parenting difficulties that are linked to daughters' HIV risk. The answers to these questions will help inform the potential development of interventions for strengthening parenting practices among women with histories of CSA and for reducing HIV risk in the next generation of women.

REFERENCES

Alexander, P. C., Teti, L., & Anderson, C. L. (2000). Childhood sexual abuse history and role reversal in parenting. *Child Abuse & Neglect, 24*, 829–838.

Amaro, H., Navarro, A. M., Conron, K. J., & Raj, A. (2002). Cultural influences on women's sexual health. In G. M. Wingood & R. J. DiClemente (Eds.), *Handbook of women's sexual and reproductive health* (pp. 71–92). New York: Kluwer Academic/Plenum.

Armsworth, M. W., & Stronck, K. (1999). Intergenerational effects of incest on parenting: Skills, abilities, and attitudes. *Journal of Counseling & Development, 77*, 303–314.

Arriola, K. R., Louden, T., Doldren, M. A., & Fortenberry, R. M. (2005). A meta-analysis of the relationship of child sexual abuse to HIV risk behavior among women. *Child Abuse & Neglect, 29*, 725–746.

Banyard, V. L. (1997). The impact of childhood sexual abuse and family functioning on four dimensions of women's later parenting. *Child Abuse & Neglect, 21*, 1095–1107.

Battle, C. L., Shea, M. T., Johnson, D. M., Yen, S., Zlotnick, C., Zanarini, M. C., et al. (2004). Childhood maltreatment associated with adult personality disorders: Findings from the Collaborative Longitudinal Personality Disorders Study. *Journal of Personality Disorders, 18*(2), 193–211.

Briere, J., & Runtz, M. (1988). Symptomatology associated with childhood sexual victimization in a nonclinical adult sample. *Child Abuse & Neglect, 12*, 51–59.

Brown, L. K., Lourie, K. J., Zlotnick, C., & Cohn, J. (2000). Impact of sexual abuse on the HIV-risk-related behavior of adolescents in intensive psychiatric treatment. *American Journal of Psychiatry, 157*, 1413–1415.

Browne, A., & Finkelhor, D. (1986). Impact of child sexual abuse: A review of the research. *Psychological Bulletin, 99*, 66–77.

Burkett, L. P. (1991). Parenting behaviors of women who were sexually abused as children in their families of origin. *Family Process, 30*, 421–434.

Charuvastra, A., & Cloitre, M. (2008). Social bonds and posttraumatic stress disorder. *Annual Review of Psychology, 59*, 301–328.

Classen, C. C., Palesh, O. G., & Aggarwal, R. (2005). Sexual revictimization: A review of the empirical literature. *Trauma, Violence, & Abuse, 6*(2), 103–129.

Cohen, T. (1995). Motherhood among incest survivors. *Child Abuse & Neglect, 19*, 1423–1429.

Coker, A. L. (2007). Does physical intimate partner violence affect sexual health? A systematic review. *Trauma, Violence, & Abuse, 8*(2), 149–177.

Collin-Vezina, D., Cyr, M., Pauze, R., & McDuff, P. (2005). The role of depression and dissociation in the link between childhood sexual abuse and later parental practices. *Journal of Trauma & Dissociation, 6*(1), 71–97.

Crosby, R. A., DiClemente, R. J., Wingood, G. M., Lang, D. L., & Harrington, K. (2003). Infrequent parental monitoring predicts sexually transmitted infections among low-income African American female adolescents. *Archives of Pediatrics & Adolescent Medicine, 157*, 169–173.

Crosby, R. A., & Miller, K. S. (2002). Family influences on adolescent females' sexual health. In G. M. Wingood & R. J. DiClemente (Eds.), *Handbook of women's sexual and reproductive health* (pp. 113–127). New York: Kluwer Academic/Plenum.

Crosby, R. A., Voisin, D., Salazar, L. F., DiClemente, R. J., Yarber, W. L., & Caliendo, A. M. (2006). Family influences and biologically confirmed sexually transmitted infections among detained adolescents. *American Journal of Orthopsychiatry, 76*, 389–394.

Cross, W. (2001). A personal history of childhood sexual abuse: Parenting patterns and problems. *Clinical Child Psychology and Psychiatry, 6*, 563–574.

Desjardins, J., Zelenski, J. M., & Coplan, R. J. (2008). An investigation of maternal personality, parenting styles, and subjective well-being. *Personality and Individual Differences, 44*, 587–597.

DiClemente, R. J., Wingood, G. M., Crosby, R., Sionean, C., Cobb, B. K., Harrington, K., et al. (2001). Parental monitoring: Association with adolescents' risk behaviors. *Pediatrics, 107*, 1363–1368.

DiLillo, D. (2001). Interpersonal functioning among women reporting a history of childhood sexual abuse: Empirical findings and methodological issues. *Clinical Psychology Review, 21*, 553–576.

DiLillo, D., & Damashek, A. (2003). Parenting characteristics of women reporting a history of childhood sexual abuse. *Child Maltreatment, 8*, 319–333.

Dishion, T. J., & McMahon, R. J. (1998). Parental monitoring and the prevention of child and adolescent problem behavior: A conceptual and empirical formulation. *Clinical Child & Family Psychology Review, 1*(1), 61–75.

Dittus, P. J., & Jaccard, J. (2000). Adolescents' perceptions of maternal disapproval of sex: Relationship to sexual outcomes. *Journal of Adolescent Health, 26*(4), 268–278.

Donenberg, G. R., & Pao, M. (2005). Youths and HIV/AIDS: Psychiatry's role in a changing epidemic. *Journal of the American Academy of Child & Adolescent Psychiatry, 44*, 728–747.

Dong, M., Anda, R. F., Dube, S. R., Giles, W. H., & Felitti, V. J. (2003). The relationship of exposure to childhood sexual abuse to other forms of abuse, neglect, and household dysfunction during childhood. *Child Abuse & Neglect, 27*, 625–639.

Dutra, R., Miller, K. S., & Forehand, R. (1999). The process and content of sexual communication with adolescents in two-parent families: Associations with sexual risk-taking behavior. *AIDS and Behavior, 3*(1), 59–66.

El-Bassel, N., Gilbert, L., Krishnan, S., Schilling, R. F., Gaeta, T., Purpura, S., et al. (1998). Partner violence and sexual HIV-risk behaviors among women in an inner-city emergency department. *Violence and Victims, 13*, 377–393.

Feerick, M. M., Haugaard, J. J., & Hien, D. A. (2002). Child maltreatment and adult-hood violence: The contribution of attachment and drug abuse. *Child Maltreatment, 7*, 226–240.

Feiring, C., & Taska, L. S. (2005). The persistence of shame following sexual abuse: A longitudinal look at risk and recovery. *Child Maltreatment, 10*, 337–349.

Fergusson, D. M., Horwood, L., & Lynskey, M. T. (1996). Childhood sexual abuse and psychiatric disorder in young adulthood: II. Psychiatric outcomes of childhood sexual abuse. *Journal of the American Academy of Child & Adolescent Psychiatry, 35*, 1365–1374.

Fergusson, D. M., Lynskey, M. T., & Horwood, L. (1996). Childhood sexual abuse and psychiatric disorder in young adulthood: I. Prevalence of sexual abuse and factors associated with sexual abuse. *Journal of the American Academy of Child & Adolescent Psychiatry, 35*, 1355–1364.

Finkelhor, D., & Browne, A. (1985). The traumatic impact of child sexual abuse: A conceptualization. *American Journal of Orthopsychiatry, 55*, 530–541.

Fossati, A., Madeddu, F., & Maffei, C. (1999). Borderline personality disorder and childhood sexual abuse: A meta-analytic study. *Journal of Personality Disorders, 13*(3), 268–280.

Henrich, C. C., Brookmeyer, K. A., Shrier, L. A., & Shahar, G. (2006). Supportive relationships and sexual risk behavior in adolescence: An ecological-transactional approach. *Journal of Pediatric Psychology, 31*, 286–297.

Hiebert-Murphy, D., & Richert, M. (2000). A parenting group for women dealing with child sexual abuse and substance abuse. *International Journal of Group Psychotherapy, 50*, 397–405.

Hutchinson, M. (2002). The influence of sexual risk communication between parents and daughters on sexual risk behaviors. *Family Relations, 51*(3), 238–247.

Hutchinson, M., Jemmott, J. B., III, Jemmott, L. S., Braverman, P., & Fong, G. T. (2003). The role of mother-daughter sexual risk communication in reducing sexual risk behaviors among urban adolescent females: A prospective study. *Journal of Adolescent Health, 33*(2), 98–107.

Johnsen, L. W., & Harlow, L. L. (1996). Childhood sexual abuse linked with adult substance use, victimization, and AIDS risk. *AIDS Education and Prevention, 8*(1), 44–57.

Kotchick, B. A., Dorsey, S., Miller, K. S., & Forehand, R. (1999). Adolescent sexual risk-taking behavior in single-parent ethnic minority families. *Journal of Family Psychology, 13*(1), 93–102.

Kotchick, B. A., Shaffer, A., & Forehand, R. (2001). Adolescent sexual risk behavior: A multi-system perspective. *Clinical Psychology Review, 21*, 493–519.

Loeb, T. B., Williams, J. K., Carmona, J. V., Rivkin, I., Wyatt, G. E., Chin, D., et al. (2002). Child sexual abuse: Associations with the sexual functioning of adolescents and adults. *Annual Review of Sex Research, 13*, 307–345.

Logan, T. K., Cole, J., & Leukefeld, C. (2002). Women, sex, and HIV: Social and contextual factors, meta-analysis of published interventions, and implications for practice and research. *Psychological Bulletin, 128*, 851–885.

Luster, T., & Small, S. A. (1994). Factors associated with sexual risk-taking behaviors among adolescents. *Journal of Marriage and Family, 56*, 622–632.

Maker, A. H., & Buttenheim, M. (2000). Parenting difficulties in sexual-abuse survivors: A theoretical framework with dual psychodynamic and cognitive-behavioral strategies for intervention. *Psychotherapy: Theory, Research, Practice, Training, 37*(2), 159–170.

Malow, R., Devieux, J., & Lucenko, B. A. (2006). History of childhood sexual abuse as a risk factor for HIV risk behavior. *Journal of Psychological Trauma, 5*(3), 13–32.

McCloskey, L. A., & Bailey, J. A. (2000). The intergenerational transmission of risk for child sexual abuse. *Journal of Interpersonal Violence, 15*, 1019–1035.

Meneses, L. M., Orrell-Valente, J. K., Guendelman, S. R., Oman, D., & Irwin, C. E., Jr. (2006). Racial/ethnic differences in mother-daughter communication about sex. *Journal of Adolescent Health, 39*(1), 128–131.

Meston, C. M., Heiman, J. R., & Trapnell, P. D. (1999). The relation between early abuse and adult sexuality. *Journal of Sex Research, 36*, 385–395.

Meston, C. M., Rellini, A. H., & Heiman, J. R. (2006). Women's history of sexual abuse, their sexuality, and sexual self-schemas. *Journal of Consulting and Clinical Psychology, 74*, 229–236.

Miller, K. S., Fasula, A. M., Dittus, P., Wiegand, R. E., Wyckoff, S. C., & McNair, L. (in press). Barriers and facilitators to maternal communication with preadolescents about age-relevant sexual topics. *AIDS and Behavior*. Epub ahead of print. Retrieved March 6, 2009, from http://www.springerlink.com/content/f654426322832196/fulltext.pdf

Miller, M. (1999). A model to explain the relationship between sexual abuse and HIV risk among women. *AIDS Care, 11*(1), 3–20.

Molnar, B. E., Buka, S. L., & Kessler, R. C. (2001). Child sexual abuse and subsequent psychopathology: Results from the National Comorbidity Survey. *American Journal of Public Health, 91*, 753–760.

Oldham, J. M., Skodol, A. E., Kellman, H. D., Hyler, S. E., Doidge, N., Rosnick, L., et al. (1995). Comorbidity of Axis I and Axis II disorders. *American Journal of Psychiatry, 152*, 571–578.

Riggs, S. A., Sahl, G., Greenwald, E., Atkison, H., Paulson, A., & Ross, C. A. (2007). Family environment and adult attachment as predictors of psychopathology and personality dysfunction among inpatient abuse survivors. *Violence and Victims, 22*, 577–600.

Risser, H. J., Hetzel-Riggin, M. D., Thomsen, C. J., & McCanne, T. R. (2006). PTSD as a mediator of sexual revictimization: The role of reexperiencing, avoidance, and arousal Symptoms. *Journal of Traumatic Stress, 19*, 687–698.

Roberts, R., O'Connor, T., Dunn, J., & Golding, J. (2004). The effects of child sexual abuse in later family life; mental health, parenting and adjustment of offspring. *Child Abuse & Neglect, 28*, 525–545.

Rodgers, K. B. (1999). Parenting processes related to sexual risk-taking behaviors of adolescent males and females. *Journal of Marriage and Family, 61*, 99–109.

Rodriguez, N., Vande Kemp, H., & Foy, D. W. (1998). Posttraumatic stress disorder in survivors of childhood sexual and physical abuse: A critical review of the empirical research. *Journal of Child Sexual Abuse, 7*, 17–45.

Ruscio, A. M. (2001). Predicting the child-rearing practices of mothers sexually abused in childhood. *Child Abuse & Neglect, 25*, 369–387.

Russell, D. E. (1983). The incidence and prevalence of intrafamilial and extrafamilial sexual abuse of female children. *Child Abuse & Neglect, 7*, 133–146.

Samper, R. E., Taft, C. T., King, D. W., & King, L. A. (2004). Posttraumatic stress disorder symptoms and parenting satisfaction among a national sample of male Vietnam veterans. *Journal of Traumatic Stress, 17*, 311–315.

Schechter, D. S., Coots, T., Zeanah, C. H., Davies, M., Coates, S. W., Trabka, K. A., et al. (2005). Maternal mental representations of the child in an inner-city clinical sample: Violence-related posttraumatic stress and reflective functioning. *Attachment & Human Development, 7*(3), 313–331.

Schechter, D. S., Zygmunt, A., Coates, S. W., Davies, M., Trabka, K. A., McCaw, J., et al. (2007). Caregiver traumatization adversely impacts young children's mental representations on the MacArthur Story Stem Battery. *Attachment & Human Development, 9*(3), 187–205.

Schuetze, P., & Eiden, R. D. (2005). The relationship between sexual abuse during childhood and parenting outcomes: Modeling direct and indirect pathways. *Child Abuse & Neglect, 29*, 645–659.

Senn, T. E., Carey, M. P., & Vanable, P. A. (2008). Childhood and adolescent sexual abuse and subsequent sexual risk behavior: Evidence from controlled studies, methodological critique, and suggestions for research. *Clinical Psychology Review, 28*, 711–735.

Senn, T. E., Carey, M. P., Vanable, P. A., Coury-Doniger, P., & Urban, M. A. (2006). Childhood sexual abuse and sexual risk behavior among men and women attending a sexually transmitted disease clinic. *Journal of Consulting and Clinical Psychology, 74*, 720–731.

Senn, T. E., Carey, M. P., Vanable, P. A., Coury-Doniger, P., & Urban, M. (2007). Characteristics of sexual abuse in childhood and adolescence influence sexual risk behavior in adulthood. *Archives of Sexual Behavior, 36*, 637–645.

Sidebotham, P., Golding, J., & the Alspac Study Team. (2001). Child maltreatment in the "children of the nineties": A longitudinal study of parental risk factors. *Child Abuse & Neglect, 25*, 1177–1200.

Simpson, T. L., & Miller, W. R. (2002). Concomitance between childhood sexual and physical abuse and substance use problems: A review. *Clinical Psychology Review, 22*, 27–77.

Smith, C. L., Spinrad, T. L., Eisenberg, N., Gaertner, B. M., Popp, T. K., & Maxon, E. (2007). Maternal personality: Longitudinal associations to parenting behavior and maternal emotional expressions toward toddlers. *Parenting: Science and Practice, 7*(3), 305–329.

Stattin, H., & Kerr, M. (2000). Parental monitoring: A reinterpretation. *Child Development, 71*, 1072–1085.

Substance Abuse and Mental Health Services Administration. (2006). *Results from the 2005 National Survey on Drug Use and Health: National findings* (DHHS

Publication No. SMA 06-4194). Rockville, MD: U.S. Department of Health and Human Services.

Sullivan, T. P., Cavanaugh, C. E., Ufner, M. J., Swan, S. C., & Snow, D. L. (in press). Relationships among women's use of aggression, their victimization and substance use problems: A test of the moderating effects of race/ethnicity. *Journal of Aggression, Maltreatment & Trauma.*

Trobst, K. K., Herbst, J. H., Masters, H. L., & Costa, P. T., Jr. (2002). Personality pathways to unsafe sex: Personality, condom use and HIV risk behaviors. *Journal of Research in Personality, 36*(2), 117–133.

U.S. Department of Justice, Office of Justice Programs, and Bureau of Justice Statistics. (2007). *Intimate partner violence in the U.S.: Victim characteristics.* Retrieved March 17, 2008, from www.ojp.usdoj.gov/bjs/intimate/victims.htm#race

Usher-Seriki, K. K., Smith Bynum, M., & Callands, T. A. (2008). Mother-daughter communication about sex and sexual intercourse among middle- to upper-class African American girls. *Journal of Family Issues, 29*, 901–917.

Voisin, D. R. (2005). The relationship between violence exposure and HIV sexual risk behavior: Does gender matter? *American Journal of Orthopsychiatry, 75*, 497–506.

Weiss, E. L., Longhurst, J. G., & Mazure, C. M. (1999). Childhood sexual abuse as a risk factor for depression in women: Psychosocial and neurobiological correlates. *American Journal of Psychiatry, 156*, 816–828.

Whitbeck, L. B., Simons, R. L., & Kao, M. (1994). The effects of divorced mothers' dating behaviors and sexual attitudes on the sexual attitudes and behaviors of their adolescent children. *Journal of Marriage and Family, 56*, 615–621.

Wingood, G. M., & DiClemente, R. J. (2000). Application of the theory of gender and power to examine HIV-related exposures, risk factors, and effective interventions for women. *Health Education & Behavior, 27*, 539–565.

Wyatt, G. E., Carmona, J. V., Loeb, T. B., Ayala, A., & Chin, D. (2002). Sexual abuse. In G. M. Wingood & R. J. DiClemente (Eds.), *Handbook of women's sexual and reproductive health* (pp. 195–216). New York: Kluwer Academic/Plenum.

Wyatt, G. E., Loeb, T. B., Solis, B., Carmona, J. V., & Romero, G. (1999). The prevalence and circumstances of child sexual abuse: Changes across a decade. *Child Abuse & Neglect, 23*, 45–60.

A Review of Childhood Abuse, Health, and Pain-Related Problems: The Role of Psychiatric Disorders and Current Life Stress

NATALIE SACHS-ERICSSON, PhD, KIARA CROMER, MS,
and ANNYA HERNANDEZ, MS

Department of Psychology, Florida State University, Tallahassee, Florida, USA

KATHLEEN KENDALL-TACKETT, PhD

Department of Pediatrics, Texas Tech University School of Medicine, Amarillo, Texas, USA

The current article reviews recent research demonstrating the relationship between childhood physical and sexual abuse and adult health problems. Adult survivors of childhood abuse have more health problems and more painful symptoms. We have found that psychiatric disorders account for some, but not all, of these symptoms, and that current life stress doubles the effect of childhood abuse on health problems. Possible etiologic factors in survivors' health problems include abuse-related alterations in brain functioning that can increase vulnerability to stress and decrease immune function. Adult survivors are also more likely to participate in risky behaviors that undermine health or to have cognitions and beliefs that amplify health problems. Psychiatric disorders, although not the primary cause of difficulties, do have a role in exacerbating health and pain-related problems. We conclude by outlining treatment recommendations for abuse survivors in health care settings.

Over the past decade, researchers have documented the relationship between childhood abuse and a number of serious health problems. The initial studies, which collected data primarily from samples of women seeking medical treatment, noted that adult survivors of childhood abuse had more medical problems than their nonabused counterparts (Sachs-Ericsson, Blazer, Plant, & Arnow, 2005). These medical problems included diabetes (Kendall-Tackett & Marshall, 1999), gastrointestinal problems (Drossman, Talley, Leserman, Olden, & Barreiro, 1995; Leserman, 2005), and obesity (Williamson, Thompson, Anda, Dietz, & Felitti, 2002). Abuse has been related to gynecological problems, headaches, arthritis, and breast cancer for women (Golding, 1994, 1999; Golding, Wilsnack, & Learman, 1998; Stein & Barrett-Connor, 2000) and thyroid disease for men (Stein & Barrett-Connor, 2000). Furthermore, childhood sexual abuse has been found to be associated with chronic fatigue, bladder problems, asthma, and heart problems, including ischemic heart disease (Dong et al., 2004; Romans, Belaise, Martin, Morris, & Raffi, 2002). Not surprisingly, abuse survivors also use more health care services (Biggs, Aziz, Tomenson, & Creed, 2003; Finestone et al., 2000).

Findings from epidemiological studies have been similar. For example, Golding and colleagues found that lifetime sexual abuse negatively impacts women's overall health (Golding, 1994, 2003; Golding, Cooper, & George, 1997). Similarly, Thompson, Kingree, and Desai (2004) found that childhood physical abuse increased health problems for men and women. A nationally representative survey of adults noted an increased odds ratio of gastrointestinal problems and migraine headaches for survivors of physical abuse (Goodwin, Hoven, Murison, & Hotopf, 2003). Researchers in a large Canadian study (Chartier, Walker, & Naimark, 2007) also found a moderate association between childhood abuse and multiple health problems, poor or fair self-rated health, pain that interferes with activities, disability due to physical health problems, and frequent emergency department and health professional visits.

Using data from the National Comorbidity Survey (NCS; Sachs-Ericsson et al., 2005), we found that childhood sexual and physical abuse increased prevalence of serious health problems for both men and women, even after we controlled for current psychiatric problems and family-of-origin issues, such as family-of-origin income, early parental loss, and parental psychiatric problems. Individuals who had been either sexually or physically abused were 1.5 to 2 times more likely to have a serious health problem than their nonabused counterparts. After controlling for the influence of family-of-origin variables and participants' current psychiatric diagnoses, we found that the relationship between childhood abuse and several health problems remained significant. These problems included blindness or deafness; heart problems; and lupus, thyroid, or autoimmune problems (Cromer & Sachs-Ericsson, 2006).

ABUSE AND CHRONIC PAIN SYNDROMES

In clinical settings, abuse survivors report more chronic pain (Kendall-Tackett, 2001), including generalized pain (Finestone et al., 2000; C. Green,

Flowe-Valencia, Rosenblum, & Tait, 2001; Kendall-Tackett, 2001; Kendall-Tackett, Marshall, & Ness, 2003), pelvic pain and vulvodynia (Harlow & Stewart, 2005; Lampe et al., 2003; Latthe, Mignini, Gray, Hills, & Khan, 2006), fibromyalgia (Boisset-Pioro, Esdaile, & Fitzcharles, 1995), chronic musculoskeletal pain (Kopec & Sayre, 2004), headache (Golding, 1999), and irritable bowel syndrome and gastrointestinal illnesses (Drossman et al., 2000; Leserman, 2005; Leserman et al., 1996; Talley, Fett, & Zinsmeister, 1995). Similarly, epidemiological studies have documented that several painful medical conditions (e.g., painful gynecological problems, headaches, arthritis, musculature pain, tender-point pain, back pain, and generally distressing physical symptoms) are more common among abuse survivors (Golding, 1994, 1999; Goodwin et al., 2003; Linton, 2002; McBeth, Macfarlane, Benjamin, Morris, & Silman, 1999; Romans et al., 2002).

In our research with the NCS sample, we examined a wide range of medical problems and the degree of reported pain associated with each of these conditions, and we compared individuals with a history of physical or sexual abuse to those with no abuse history. We found that individuals who experienced abuse reported more pain in relation to their current health problems than those without abuse experiences (Sachs-Ericsson, Kendall-Tackett, & Hernandez, 2007).

ADDITIVE AFFECT OF ABUSE EXPERIENCES AND OTHER CHILDHOOD ADVERSITIES

Children who experience one type of abuse are likely to experience other types. For example, Felitti and colleagues (1998) found that when respondents experienced one type of childhood adversity, the probability of having experienced another was approximately 80. Unfortunately, experiencing more than one type of childhood abuse compounds the effects, leading to even poorer health outcomes (e.g., Arnow, Hart, Hayward, Dea, & Barr Taylor, 2000; Diaz, Simantov, & Rickert, 2000; Felitti et al., 1998; Golding et al., 1997; Kessler, 2000; Kessler, Davis, & Kendler, 1997; Thompson, Arias, Basile, & Desai, 2002; Walker et al., 1999). Kessler argued that researchers often look at one type of childhood adversity, such as physical abuse, and assume subsequent problems are related to that, ignoring the possibility that physical abuse often co-occurs within a cluster of other childhood difficulties that may account for the symptoms they see. More recently, Finkelhor, Ormrod, and Turner (2007) found that poly-victimization was more likely to predict trauma symptoms than a single type of victimization.

Researchers have documented the fact that family characteristics associated with childhood abuse can also contribute to the development of subsequent health-related problems. These include parental psychopathology, family conflict, low socioeconomic status, parental loss or absence, and parental divorce (Felitti et al., 1998; Fleming, Mullen, & Bammer, 1997; Kenny & McEachern, 2000; Molnar, Buka, & Kessler, 2001; Romans, Martin, Anderson, O'Shea, & Mullen, 1995; Sidebotham, Golding, & the ALSPAC Study Team, 2001; Zuravin & Fontanella, 1999). In order to understand the implications of each type of specific childhood abuse adversity on health, it is important for researchers to try to distinguish the influence of each from other co-occurring childhood adversities.

In our work, we found that several family-of-origin variables were clearly associated with adult health problems (Sachs-Ericsson et al., 2005). Specifically, parents' psychiatric disorders, parental abandonment, parental divorce, low levels of parental education, and family conflict were all associated with subsequent health problems in adults. However, even after we controlled for these family-of-origin factors, there remained a significant relationship between childhood abuse and health status, with abuse survivors reporting more health problems and pain. Thus, our work supports the conclusion that childhood sexual and physical abuse have an effect on adult health problems and pain reports above and beyond family-of-origin factors.

WHY CHILD ABUSE MAKES PEOPLE SICK: ETIOLOGICAL PATHWAYS BETWEEN ABUSE AND HEALTH OUTCOMES

As we described in the section above, childhood abuse can have major negative effects on health. The intriguing question then becomes this: Why is this so? Why does child abuse make people sick? Early abuse experiences may have an impact on adult health outcomes via several pathways (Kendall-Tackett, 2003). Direct injury is the most obvious way that abuse could be related to health, but it does not account for all health effects (Leserman et al., 1997). For example, sexual abuse may also result in sexually transmitted diseases (Hillis, Anda, Felitti, Nordenberg, & Marchbanks, 2000) or unwanted pregnancy (Dietz et al., 1999), which may lead to subsequent health problems in adulthood. Similarly, physical abuse can lead to physical injuries, including traumatic brain injury (Banks, 2007).

Behavior can also impact health. Abuse survivors, as well as persons who have experienced other types of childhood adversities, are more likely to participate in high-risk behaviors (Kendall-Tackett, 2002, 2003). Most of these behaviors and problems are associated with the leading causes of morbidity and mortality in the United States (Anderson, Kochanek, & Murphy, 1997). For example, abuse survivors are more likely to abuse substances, drive while intoxicated, smoke, compulsively overeat, be severely obese, avoid exercise, and engage in risky sexual behavior (Felitti et al., 1998; Fleming, Mullen, Sibthorpe, & Bammer, 1999; Kaplan et al., 1998; Nichols & Harlow, 2004; Springs & Friedrich, 1992; Walker et al., 1999; Williamson et al., 2002).

Moreover, childhood abuse may increase the risk of health problems through comorbid psychiatric disorders and the impact of early abuse experiences on the developing brain. Early life stress has been found to influence immune functioning and sensitivity to stress, which may in turn contribute to increased health problems. Problems related to psychiatric disorders include low self-esteem, poor coping skills, disturbed self-identity, poor interpersonal skills, insecure attachment styles, and increased vulnerability to stress (Becker-Lausen & Mallon-Kraft, 1997; Romans et al., 2002; Waldinger, Schulz, Barsky, & Ahern, 2006). Individuals with a history of sexual assault were found to have less contact with and to have received less support from friends and family (Golding, Wilsnack, & Cooper, 2002). Social support, in turn, has repeatedly been shown to be a major protective factor against psychiatric disorders, particularly depression (Plant & Sachs-Ericsson, 2004), and has also been shown to influence health outcomes (Israel, Farquhar, Schulz, James, & Parker, 2002; Lett et al., 2005).

Early Abuse, Stress, and the Developing Brain

Abuse experiences may also result in physiological alterations, including changes in the developing brain (Heim & Nemeroff, 2002; Kendall-Tackett, 2002, 2003). These trauma-related changes can contribute to increased physiological reactivity to current stressors. For example, Thakkar and McCanne (2000) found that women with a history of abuse reported more physical symptoms in response to daily stress than women with no abuse history.

Another physiologic sequela of early life stress is enhanced sensitivity of the hypothalamic–pituitary–adrenal axis (Kendall-Tackett, 2002). These alterations have been observed in individuals with posttraumatic stress disorder (PTSD) and women who have experienced childhood sexual abuse (Yehuda, Boisoneau, Lowy, & Giller, 1995). Ongoing activation of the hypothalamic–pituitary–adrenal axis may result in an individual having abnormally low levels of cortisol or becoming cortisol resistant (Kendall-Tackett, 2008). In either case, immune function is impaired, increasing the chance of illness (Altemus, Cloitre, & Dhabhar, 2003; Heim & Nemeroff, 2002).

Abuse, Stress Reactivity, and the Immune System

In our research, we found that current stressful life events moderated the relationship between childhood abuse and adult health problems. Specifically, the presence of stress more than doubled the effect of physical or sexual abuse on health problems (Cromer & Sachs-Ericsson, 2006). Our findings are consistent with past research on the relationship between childhood abuse and the sensitization of stress-responsive neurobiological systems. Childhood abuse can also dysregulate the immune system, which can increase psychiatric morbidity among individuals with abuse histories. Specifically, individuals with PTSD (resulting from childhood sexual abuse) displayed several markers of increased immune activation (Wilson, Calhoun, & Bernat, 1999). Moreover, depression, which is highly comorbid with childhood abuse, has also been associated with impaired immune functioning, with increased cytokine secretion, and with dysregulation of cortisol, implicated as mechanisms by which the immune system becomes less effective (Connor & Leonard, 1998; Kendall-Tackett, 2008; Maes, Bosmans, & Meltzer, 1995). This paradigm of immune dysregulation among individuals with childhood abuse is consistent with research findings that indicate that autoimmune problems are more frequent in individuals with a history of childhood abuse (Dallam, 2005). Thus, it seems that immunological research, in conjunction with research on childhood abuse, is a promising area for future investigation.

The Role of Psychiatric Disorders in Health Outcomes

What is the role of psychiatric disorders in adult survivors' health symptoms? Abuse survivors have higher rates of psychiatric problems (e.g., Kendler et al., 2000), which has been found to be related to health status (e.g., Schnurr & Spiro, 1999). Indeed, some have hypothesized that psychiatric problems may mediate the influence of childhood abuse on health problems (Golding, 1994; Verona & Sachs-Ericsson, 2005). However, several studies have found that the influence has been relatively minimal. For example, in their meta-analysis, Golding and colleagues (1997) concluded that depression did not markedly change the influence of abuse on subjective health. Nor did psychiatric disorders mediate the association between child abuse and pain reports (Walsh, Jamieson, MacMillan, & Boyle, 2007). In our research with the NCS sample, we found that lifetime psychiatric disorders partially mediated the relationship between abuse and the occurrence of the 1-year prevalence of serious health problems, but the effects were relatively minimal. Nonetheless, our work with the NCS data has shown that psychiatric disorders contribute to the relationship between abuse and health (Sachs-Ericsson et al., 2005, 2007).

The Mechanism Underlying Abuse and Pain Sensitivity

Abuse survivors also report experiencing more pain in relation to their health problems (Sachs-Ericsson, Verona, Joiner, & Preacher, 2006). Several theories have been put forth to account for increased pain in abuse survivors. Childhood abuse may contribute to a negative attributional style (Sachs-Ericsson et al., 2006), an inability to manage stress (Kendall-Tackett, 2001), and limited social support (Golding et al., 2002)—each of which may exacerbate pain. Researchers have suggested that trauma-related alterations in neurosensory processing may amplify pain (Arnow et al., 2000; Drossman, 1994), and child-hood abuse lowers pain thresholds (Scarinci, McDonald-Haile, Bradley, & Richter, 1994).

What is interesting is that results of an experimental study suggested that individuals with a history of childhood abuse may have a decreased sensitivity to experimentally induced pain; however, these individuals also had more difficulties related to chronic pain. As the authors noted, their findings highlight the complexity of the relationship between abuse history and pain, thereby illustrating the need for further investigation of pain-related correlates of abuse (Fillingim & Edwards, 2005).

Some of this increased pain may be due to depression. Depression is common among adult survivors of abuse (Goldberg, 1994; Levitan et al., 1998; Molnar et al., 2001; Roosa, Reinholtz, & Angelini, 1999; Turner & Muller, 2004; Zuravin & Fontanella, 1999) and among patients with chronic pain (Faucett, 1994; Fishbain, Cutler, Rosomoff, & Rosomoff, 1997; Magni, Moreschi, Rigatti-Luchini, & Merskey, 1994; McWilliams, Cox, & Enns, 2003). Moreover, past research has shown that depression increases pain reports among individuals with health problems (Hernandez & Sachs-Ericsson, 2006).

From a physiological standpoint, pain and depression are quite similar and may, in fact, become mutually maintaining conditions (Meagher, 2004). Specifically, depression is associated with a neurochemical imbalance of neurotransmitters (Bair, Robinson, Katon, & Kroenke, 2003; Fava, 2003), including serotonin, norepinephrine, and dopamine (Andrews & Pinder, 2000; Blackburn-Munro & Blackburn-Munro, 2001). Analgesic effects are pro-duced by serotonin and norepinephrine through descending pain pathways, and these effects may be disrupted by decreased levels of these neurotrans-mitters (Andrews & Pinder, 2000). The pain modulation system influences affect and attention to peripheral stimuli and plays a role in suppressing minor signals coming from the body (Blackburn-Munro & Blackburn-Munro, 2001; Stahl, 2002). These signals may be less suppressed when serotonin and norepinephrine are depleted (Bair et al., 2003). Thus, the association between pain and depression may be due, in part, to the neurochemical impact depression plays in the pain response (Blackburn-Munro & Blackburn-Munro, 2001).

Emotionally negative mood states may also reduce tolerance to aversive stimuli (Meagher, Arnau, & Rhudy, 2001; Zelman, Howland, Nichols, & Cleeland, 1991). The motivational priming model proposes that negative emotional states enhance pain perception, whereas pleasant affective states attenuate it. Specifically, studies have shown that negative affect decreased pain tolerance to aversive stimuli whereas positive affect increased tolerance to aversive stimuli (Meagher et al., 2001; Zelman et al., 1991). Thus, negative emotions seem to magnify patients' experiences of pain.

Abuse, pain, and depression. In our research, abuse survivors reported more pain in relation to their health problems than did their nonabused counterparts (Sachs-Ericsson et al., 2007). We also hypothesized that because childhood abuse is associated with higher rates of depression, and depression is associated with more reported pain, depression would mediate the relationship between childhood abuse and adult pain reports. Indeed, we did find higher rates of pain and higher rates of depression among abuse survivors. We initially found that depression did mediate the relationship between childhood abuse and pain reports. However, after we controlled for differences between abused and nonabused participants on specific health problems (which were greater among the abused participants), depression did not mediate the relationship. Thus, we concluded that the higher rate of depression found among abuse survivors was not the primary factor for their increased pain reports. Rather, childhood abuse and depression independently contributed to pain reports (Sachs-Ericsson et al., 2007). Thus, both depression and pain, common sequelae of childhood abuse, need to be appropriately addressed within the context of medical and psychological treatments.

TREATMENT IMPLICATIONS

This review has highlighted the connection between childhood abuse and poor health in adult survivors. The ongoing costs of childhood abuse—both personal and societal—are enormous and provide the impetus for understanding the mechanisms by which events in childhood can lead to poor health (Schnurr & Green, 2004). The first step in attenuating the physical health consequences of abuse is to identify abuse survivors when they present in medical or mental health settings (Schnurr & Green, 2004). From a mind–body perspective, the accurate diagnosis of both physical and mental illnesses is a key step in improving a patient's overall health. Mental health professionals need to consider both the patient's physical and mental health in the context of an overall treatment plan. Medical personnel also need to understand the possible health implications of an abuse history and its psychiatric sequelae (Schnurr & Green, 2004).

Universal screening for depression, with follow-up referrals, may prove to be the most cost-effective way of detecting depression in medical settings (B. L. Green & Kimmerling, 2004; Schoenbaum et al., 2001). It is also possible that similar methods could aid in the identification of other psychiatric disorders that are commonly associated with childhood abuse, such as PTSD and other anxiety disorders. Abuse survivors with chronic pain will also need an integrative approach to treatment that addresses both their physical health complaints and any depression or other psychiatric disorder that may be magnifying their symptoms. Any treatment that ignores both components will be incomplete. Screening for pain can initially be completed with the use of a one- or two-item pain measure, such as asking patients to rate their current level of pain on a scale from 0 to 10, with 0 being *no pain* and 10 being *intense pain*.

Mental health professionals must also be aware that some of their patients may be at risk for serious health problems. One helpful step may be for clinicians to assess a patient's general physical health history in conjunction with his or her mental health history. Furthermore, mental health practitioners may wish to refer their patients to a non-psychiatric physician to aid in the detection of any potential medical problems (DeVellis & DeVellis, 2001). Mental health care can be an important adjunct to medical care and should specifically address psychological and behavioral variables that may contribute to or exacerbate medically related conditions, such as risky health behaviors or catastrophizing cognitions related to physical symptoms.

Recommendations for Treatment

In health care settings, sensitivity to the needs of abuse survivors can enhance the effectiveness of their care (Monahan & Forgash, 2000; Schachter, Radomsky, Stalker, & Teram, 2004). Some issues specifically related to caring for an abuse survivor include increasing the patient's sense of safety; approaching the disclosure of childhood abuse in an open and empathic manner; and being sensitive to abuse-related issues, such as boundaries, the effects of trauma on the body, and the potential for flashback triggers. Schachter and colleagues found that a general approach is to treat the clinician–patient relationship as a collaborative partnership, which encourages patients to be more in control of deciding a treatment course. If patients are educated about their illnesses and their available treatment options, they are more likely to comply with treatment. If both patients and care providers are aware of the physical and mental health consequences of childhood abuse, then abuse survivors are more likely to receive appropriate—and effective—care.

In addition to the more general implications discussed above, there are several specific treatment guidelines and recommendations. These include monitoring health-risk behaviors and helping patients both reduce current life stress and strengthen their social support.

As we described, abuse survivors are more likely to participate in high-risk behaviors that increase their risk of illness and premature mortality (Kendall-Tackett, 2001). With regard to treatment, it is important for primary care physicians to screen and monitor these behaviors, given their connection to many medical problems. Mental health professionals should also screen and monitor these behaviors as they may represent poor coping skills used to deal with trauma-associated psychological distress (Davis, Combs-Lane, & Smith, 2004; Springs & Friedrich, 1992). These ineffective coping methods can be replaced during therapy with strategies that are healthier from both a mental and physical health standpoint. Risky health behaviors, such as smoking or substance use, are not easily addressed in treatment. Rather, they require dedicated treatment programs to increase the individual's motivation to reduce risky behaviors, develop skills for dealing with life stressors, and, just as important, directly address the psychiatric symptoms often associated with individuals who engage in risky health behaviors. Others believe that individuals who engage in risky health behaviors will make significant strides in making effective changes when they are enrolled in specialized treatments. These specialized programs target the specific needs of subgroups of individuals, such as those who experience high negative affect or those who abuse substances, rather than expect any single treatment approach to be a panacea (Brown, 2003; Shiffman, 1993).

Another specific treatment recommendation is to help abuse survivors reduce current life stress. A growing body of literature indicates that current life stress can exacerbate the relationship between trauma and poor health (e.g., Cromer & Sachs-Ericsson, 2006). Moreover, stress is an important factor in the onset and relapse of most psychiatric disorders (Rende & Plomin, 1992). Education on this relationship can empower patients, and a proportion of treatment should help abuse survivors lower their stress levels.

Yet another specific recommendation for treating abuse survivors is to strengthen their social support networks. Abuse survivors often have low levels of social support, and this can dramatically impair their health (Biggs, Aziz, Tomenson, & Creed, 2004). Supportive disclosures of assaults can act as a buffer against increased health problems (Kimerling & Calhoun, 1994), and social support is also an important buffer against psychiatric disorders, and in particular depression (Joiner, Coyne, & Haslam, 2000; Petty, Sachs-Ericsson, & Joiner, 2004). Several psychotherapy protocols focus on increasing interpersonal skills and social support, thereby reducing reactivity to stress. For example, dialectical behavior therapy focuses on building interpersonal relationships, increasing stress tolerance, and developing self-soothing behaviors (Comtois & Linehan, 2006). Exposure-based therapies, which are effective for treating anxiety disorders, help abuse survivors with health problems function more effectively (Leserman, 2005). However, as Leserman noted, the field needs more research examining psychological treatments that might be effective specifically for treating physical health problems associated with sexual abuse history.

Our research suggests that childhood abuse and depression independently contribute to pain experiences for individuals in chronic pain. If an abuse survivor has comorbid pain and depression, addressing one problem without the other would not adequately meet his or her treatment needs. Many of the same recommendations described above for increasing social skills, increasing social support networks, and decreasing stress are also applicable to the treatment of comorbid pain and depression among individuals with a history of abuse. Additionally, both depression and chronic pain can be treated with antidepressants, which will help alleviate both pain and depression. Furthermore, health and pain-related problems can be treated with exercise, physical and occupational therapy, stress management, and activity pacing. Patients' catastrophizing beliefs about their health can be addressed with the use of cognitive–behavioral psychotherapy. Indeed, our research suggests that childhood abuse directly contributes to the development of a negative attributional style (Sachs-Ericsson et al., 2006). Therapy that specifically addresses this style has been found to be helpful in reducing chronic pain (Kendall-Tackett et al., 2003).

Barriers to Care

Those seeking to provide adequate and compassionate health care for abuse survivors may face several barriers. They may lack adequate assessment tools, have limited resources, and find that discussing abuse with patients is difficult or uncomfortable. Clinicians facing these barriers may be tempted to write off patients as "difficult" without understanding the role of previous trauma and the difficulties that that history can create in the patient–provider relationship (Havig, 2008). Abuse survivors often feel quite vulnerable in health care settings, and this can lead to negative patient–provider interactions. These negative interactions can exacerbate patients' psychological and health-related problems.

In a study of sexual abuse survivors, Havig (2008) found that patients were most responsive when health care providers provided an atmosphere of openness, professionalism, sensitivity, and concern. Havig concluded that providers should initiate active and routine inquiry regarding abuse. Furthermore, providers should be prepared to listen to the experiences of survivors without revictimizing, blaming, dismissing, or judging them. This will facilitate an enhanced understanding of patient needs and provide patients with the opportunity to engage in more positive health behaviors.

As Schnurr and Green (2004) noted, the association between trauma, mental health, and medical problems has "systems" and policy implications. The above recommendations, when taken altogether, may seem daunting given the current health care system. However, in order to be their most effective, primary care practitioners and mental health clinicians need to collaborate on the delivery of care for abuse survivors. An integrated care model can more effectively accomplish the preceding treatment recommendations. This collaborative model can substantially reduce health care use, increase treatment adherence, and lead to better recovery for abuse survivors (e.g., Kimerling & Calhoun, 1994).

Conclusions and Future Research

Our research, based on a large representative epidemiological sample, has extended past research by demonstrating a relationship between childhood sexual and physical abuse and increased rates of health problems. We have found that abuse survivors also have higher rates of chronic pain. Furthermore, our work has shown that current life stressors moderate the relationship between abuse and health problems, such that stress exacerbates health problems in abuse survivors.

Whereas several researchers have speculated that abuse-related health problems may be due to psychiatric disorders, we have found that psychiatric disorders have a relatively small influence on the relationship between abuse, health problems, and pain reports. From our data, it appears that health problems, chronic pain, and psychiatric disorders are all sequelae of past abuse. That conclusion should change the way that experts approach the treatment of patients. Each of these problems needs to be addressed in treatment. Addressing one problem and not the other would likely be insufficient in adequately meeting an individual's treatment needs.

The continuing influence of childhood abuse on adult health functioning, as well as the impact of current stress, underscores the significant public health concern surrounding childhood abuse. Various mechanisms most likely underlie the association between childhood abuse and poor health. Future research that identifies and elaborates on these underlying mechanisms will play an important role in extending understanding of the negative health sequelae of childhood abuse.

REFERENCES

Altemus, M., Cloitre, M., & Dhabhar, F. S. (2003). Enhanced cellular immune response in women with PTSD related to childhood abuse. *American Journal of Psychiatry, 160*, 1705–1707.

Anderson, R. N., Kochanek, K. D., & Murphy, S. L. (1997). Report of final mortality statistics, 1995. *Monthly Vital Statistics Report, 45*(11, Suppl. 2). Hyattsville, MD: National Center for Health Statistics.

Andrews, J., & Pinder, R. (2001). Antidepressants of the future: A critical assessment of the chemistry and pharmacology of novel antidepressants in development. In B. E. Leonard (Ed.), *Antidepressants* (pp. 123–146). Boston: Birkhauser.

Arnow, B., Hart, S., Hayward, C., Dea, R., & Barr Taylor, C. (2000). Severity of child maltreatment, pain complaints and medical utilization among women. *Journal of Psychiatric Research, 34*, 413–421.

Bair, M. J., Robinson, R. L., Katon, W., & Kroenke, K. (2003). Depression and pain comorbidity: A literature review. *Archives of Internal Medicine, 163*, 2433–2445.

Banks, M. (2007). Overlooked but critical: Traumatic brain injury as a consequence of interpersonal violence. *Trauma, Violence & Abuse, 8*, 290–298.

Becker-Lausen, E., & Mallon-Kraft, S. (1997). Pandemic outcomes: The intimacy variable. In G. K. Kantor & J. S. Jasinski (Eds.), *Out of darkness: Current perspectives on family violence* (pp. 49–57). Newbury Park, CA: Sage.

Biggs, A.-M., Aziz, Q., Tomenson, B., & Creed, F. (2003). Do childhood adversity and recent social stress predict health care use in patients presenting with upper abdominal or chest pain? *Psychosomatic Medicine, 65,* 1020–1028.

Biggs, A.-M., Aziz, Q., Tomenson, B., & Creed, F. (2004). Effect of childhood adversity on health related quality of life in patients with upper abdominal or chest pain. *Gut, 53,* 180–186.

Blackburn-Munro, G., & Blackburn-Munro, R. (2001). Chronic pain, chronic stress and depression: Coincidence or consequence? *Journal of Neuroendocrinology, 13,* 1009–1023.

Boisset-Pioro, M., Esdaile, J., & Fitzcharles, M. (1995). Sexual and physical abuse in women with fibromyalgia syndrome. *Arthritis & Rheumatism, 38,* 235–241.

Brown, R. A. (2003). Comorbidity treatment. In D. B. Abrams, R. S. Niaura, R. A. Brown, K. M. Emmons, M. G. Goldstein, & P. M. Monti (Eds.), *The tobacco dependence treatment handbook: A guide to best practices* (pp. 178–229). New York: Guilford Press.

Chartier, M. J., Walker, J. R., & Naimark, B. (2007). Childhood abuse, adult health, and health care utilization: Results from a representative community sample. *American Journal of Epidemiology, 165,* 1031–1038.

Comtois, K., & Linehan, M. (2006). Psychosocial treatments of suicidal behaviors: A practice-friendly review. *Journal of Clinical Psychology, 62,* 161–170.

Connor, T. J., & Leonard, B. E. (1998). Depression, stress and immunological activation: The role of cytokines in depressive disorders. *Life Sciences, 62,* 583–606.

Cromer, K., & Sachs-Ericsson, N. (2006). The association between childhood abuse, PTSD and the occurrence of adult health problems: Moderation via current life stress. *Journal of Traumatic Stress, 19,* 967–971.

Dallam, S. J. (2005). Health issues associated with violence against women. In K. A. Kendall-Tackett (Ed.), *Handbook of women, stress & trauma* (pp. 159–180). New York: Taylor & Francis.

Davis, J. L., Combs-Lane, A. M., & Smith, D. W. (2004). Victimization and health risk behaviors: Implications for prevention programs. In K. A. Kendall-Tackett (Ed.), *Health consequences of abuse in the family: A clinical guide for evidence-based practice* (pp. 179–195). Washington, DC: American Psychological Association.

DeVellis, B. M., & DeVellis, R. F. (2001). Self-efficacy and health. In A. Baum, T. A. Evenson, & J. E. Singer (Eds.), *Handbook of health psychology.* Mahwah, NJ: Erlbaum.

Diaz, A., Simantov, E., & Rickert, V. I. (2000). Effect of abuse on health: Results of a national survey. *Archives of Pediatric Adolescent Medicine, 156,* 811–817.

Dietz, P. M., Spitz, A. M., Anda, R. F., Williamson, D. F., McMahon, P. M., Santelli, J. S., et al. (1999). Unintended pregnancy among adult women exposed to abuse or household dysfunction during their childhood. *Journal of the American Medical Association, 282,* 1359–1364.

Dong, M., Giles, W. H., Felitti, V. J., Dube, S. R., Williams, J. E., Chapman, D. P., et al. (2004). Insights into causal pathways for ischemic heart disease: Adverse Childhood Experiences Study. *Circulation, 110,* 1761–1766.

Drossman, D. A. (1994). Physical and sexual abuse and gastrointestinal illness: What is the link? *American Journal of Medicine, 97,* 105–107.

Drossman, D. A., Leserman, J., Li, Z., Keefe, F., Hu, Y. J. B., & Toomey, T. C. (2000). Effects of coping on health outcome among women with gastrointestinal disorders. *Psychosomatic Medicine, 62*, 309–317.

Drossman, D. A., Talley, N. J., Leserman, J., Olden, K. W., & Barreiro, M. A. (1995). Sexual and physical abuse and gastrointestinal illness: Review and recommendations. *Annals of Internal Medicine, 123*, 782–794.

Faucett, J. (1994). Depression in painful chronic disorders: The role of pain and conflict about pain. *Journal of Pain Symptom Management, 9*, 520–526.

Fava, M. (2003). The role of the serotonergic and noradrenergic neurotransmitter systems in the treatment of psychological and physical symptoms of depression. *Journal of Clinical Psychiatry, 64*(Suppl. 13), 26–29.

Felitti, V. J., Anda, R. F., Nordenberg, D., Williamson, D. F., Spitz, A. M., Edwards, V., et al. (1998). Relationship of childhood abuse and household dysfunction to many of the leading causes of death in adults: The Adverse Childhood Experiences (ACE) Study. *American Journal of Preventive Medicine, 14*, 245–258.

Fillingim, R., & Edwards, R. (2005). Is self-reported childhood abuse history associated with pain perception among healthy young women and men? *Clinical Journal of Pain, 21*, 387–397.

Finestone, H., Stenn, P., Davies, F., Stalker, C., Fry, R., & Koumanis, J. (2000). Chronic pain and health care utilization in women with a history of childhood sexual abuse. *Child Abuse & Neglect, 24*, 547–556.

Finkelhor, D., Ormrod, R. K., & Turner, H. A. (2007). Poly-victimization and trauma in a national longitudinal cohort. *Development and Psychopathology, 19*(1), 149–166.

Fishbain, D., Cutler, R., Rosomoff, H., & Rosomoff, R. (1997). Chronic pain-associated depression: Antecedent or consequence of chronic pain? A review. *Clinical Journal of Pain, 13*, 116–137.

Fleming, J., Mullen, P., & Bammer, G. (1997). A study of potential risk factors for sexual abuse in childhood. *Child Abuse & Neglect, 21*, 49–58.

Fleming, J., Mullen, P. E., Sibthorpe, B., & Bammer, G. (1999). The long-term impact of childhood sexual abuse in Australian women. *Child Abuse & Neglect, 23*, 145–159.

Goldberg, R. (1994). Childhood abuse, depression, and chronic pain. *Clinical Journal of Pain, 10*, 277–281.

Golding, J. M. (1994). Sexual assault history and physical health in randomly selected Los Angeles women. *Health Psychology, 13*, 130–138.

Golding, J. M. (1999). Sexual-assault history and long-term physical health problems: Evidence from clinical and population epidemiology. *Current Directions in Psychological Science, 8*(6), 191–194.

Golding, J. M. (2003). Sexual-assault history and long-term physical health problems: Evidence from clinical and population epidemiology. *Directions in Psychological Science, 8*, 191–194.

Golding, J. M., Cooper, M. L., & George, L. K. (1997). Sexual assault history and health perceptions: Seven general population studies. *Health Psychology, 16*, 417–425.

Golding, J., Wilsnack, S., & Cooper, M. (2002). Sexual assault history and social support: Six general population studies. *Journal of Traumatic Stress, 15*(3), 187–197.

Golding, J. M., Wilsnack, S. C., & Learman, L. A. (1998). Prevalence of sexual assault history among women with common gynecologic symptoms. *American Journal of Obstetrics and Gynecology, 179*, 1013–1019.

Goodwin, R. D., Hoven, C. W., Murison, R., & Hotopf, M. (2003). Association between childhood physical abuse and gastrointestinal disorders and migraine in adulthood. *American Journal of Public Health, 93*, 1065–1067.

Green, B. L., & Kimmerling, R. (2004). Trauma, posttraumatic stress disorder, and health status. In P. Schnurr & B. L. Green (Eds.), *Trauma and health: Physical health consequences of exposure in extreme stress* (pp. 129–155). Washington, DC: American Psychological Association.

Green, C., Flowe-Valencia, H., Rosenblum, L., & Tait, A. (2001). The role of childhood and adulthood abuse among women presenting for chronic pain management. *Clinical Journal of Pain, 17*, 359–364.

Harlow, B. L., & Stewart, E. G. (2005). Adult-onset vulvodynia in relation to childhood violence victimization. *American Journal of Epidemiology, 161*, 871–880.

Havig, K. (2008). The health care experiences of adult survivors of child sexual abuse: A systematic review of evidence on sensitive practice. *Trauma Violence Abuse, 9*(1), 19–33.

Heim, C., & Nemeroff, C. B. (2002). Neurobiology of early life stress: Clinical studies. *Seminar in Clinical Neuropsychiatry, 7*, 147–159.

Hernandez, A., & Sachs-Ericsson, N. (2006). Ethnic differences in pain reports and the moderating role of depression in a community sample of Hispanic and Caucasian participants with serious health problems. *Psychosomatic Medicine, 68*, 121–128.

Hillis, S. D., Anda, R. F., Felitti, V. J., Nordenberg, D., & Marchbanks, P. A. (2000). Adverse childhood experiences and sexually transmitted diseases in men and women: A retrospective study. *Pediatrics, 106*, E11.

Israel, B. A., Farquhar, S. A., Schulz, A. J., James, S. A., & Parker, E. A. (2002). The relationship between social support, stress, and health among women on Detroit's east side. *Health Education & Behavior, 29*, 342–360.

Joiner, T., Coyne, J. C., & Haslam, N. (2000). The interactional nature of depression. *Journal of Cognitive Psychotherapy, 14*, 413–415.

Kaplan, S. J., Pelcovitz, D., Salzinger, S., Weiner, M., Mandel, F. S., & Lesser, M. L. (1998). Adolescent physical abuse: Risk for adolescent psychiatric disorders. *American Journal of Psychiatry, 155*, 954–959.

Kendall-Tackett, K. (2001). Chronic pain: The next frontier in child maltreatment research. *Child Abuse & Neglect, 25*, 997–1000.

Kendall-Tackett, K. A. (2002). The health effects of childhood abuse: Four pathways by which abuse can influence health. *Child Abuse & Neglect, 26*, 715–729.

Kendall-Tackett, K. A. (2003). *Treating the lifetime health effects of childhood victimization*. Kingston, NJ: Civic Research Institute.

Kendall-Tackett, K. A. (2008). *Non-pharmacologic treatments for depression in new mothers: Omega-3s, exercise, bright light therapy, social support, psychotherapy and St. John's Wort*. Amarillo, TX: Hale Publishing.

Kendall-Tackett, K. A., & Marshall, R. (1999). Victimization and diabetes: An exploratory study. *Child Abuse & Neglect, 23*, 593–596.

Kendall-Tackett, K. A., Marshall, R., & Ness, K. E. (2003). Chronic pain syndromes and violence against women. *Women and Therapy, 26,* 45–56.

Kendler, K. S., Bulik, C. M., Silberg, J., Hettema, J. M., Myers, J., & Prescott, C. A. (2000). Childhood sexual abuse and adult psychiatric and substance use disorders in women: An epidemiological and cotwin control analysis. *Archives of General Psychiatry, 57,* 953–959.

Kenny, M. C., & McEachern, A. G. (2000). Racial, ethnic, and cultural factors of childhood sexual abuse: A selected review of the literature. *Clinical Psychology Review, 20,* 905–922.

Kessler, R. C. (2000). The long-term effects of childhood adversities on depression and other psychiatric disorders. In T. O. Harris (Ed.), *Where inner and outer worlds meet* (pp. 227–244). London: Routledge.

Kessler, R. C., Davis, C. G., & Kendler, K. S. (1997). Childhood adversity and adult psychiatric disorder in the US National Comorbidity Survey. *Psychological Medicine, 27,* 1101–1119.

Kimerling, R., & Calhoun, K. S. (1994). Somatic symptoms, social support, and treatment seeking among sexual assault victims. *Journal of Consulting and Clinical Psychology, 62,* 333–340.

Kopec, J., & Sayre, E. (2004). Traumatic experiences in childhood and the risk of arthritis: A prospective cohort study. *Canadian Journal of Public Health, 95,* 361–365.

Lampe, A., Doering, S., Rumpold, G., Soelder, E., Krismer, M., Kantner-Rumplmair, W., et al. (2003). Chronic pain syndromes and their relation to childhood abuse and stressful life events. *Journal of Psychosomatic Research, 54,* 361–367.

Latthe, P., Mignini, L., Gray, R., Hills, R., & Khan, K. (2006). Factors predisposing women to chronic pelvic pain: Systematic review. *British Medical Journal, 332,* 749–755.

Leserman, J. (2005). Sexual abuse history: Prevalence, health effects, mediators, and psychological treatment. *Psychosomatic Medicine, 67,* 906–915.

Leserman, J., Drossman, D. A., Li, Z., Toomey, T. C., Nachman, G., & Glogau, L. (1996). Sexual and physical abuse history in gastroenterology practice: How types of abuse impact health status. *Psychosomatic Medicine, 58,* 4–15.

Leserman, J., Li, Z., Drossman, D. A., Toomey, T. C., Nachman, G., & Glogau, L. (1997). Impact of sexual and physical abuse dimensions on health status: Development of an abuse severity measure. *Psychosomatic Medicine, 59,* 152–160.

Lett, H. S., Blumenthal, J. A., Babyak, M. A., Strauman, T. J., Robins, C., & Sherwood, A. (2005). Social support and coronary heart disease: Epidemiologic evidence and implications for treatment. *Psychosomatic Medicine, 67,* 869–878.

Levitan, R. D., Parikh, S. V., Lesage, A. D., Hegadoren, K. M., Adams, M., Kennedy, S. H., et al. (1998). Major depression in individuals with a history of childhood physical or sexual abuse: Relationship to neurovegetative features, mania, and gender. *American Journal of Psychiatry, 155,* 1746–1752.

Linton, S. J. (2002). A prospective study of the effects of sexual or physical abuse on back pain. *Pain, 96,* 347–351.

Maes, M., Bosmans, E., & Meltzer, H. Y. (1995). Immunoendocrine aspects of major depression. Relationships between plasma interleukin-6 and soluble interleukin-2 receptor, prolactin and cortisol. *European Archives of Psychiatry and Clinical Neuroscience, 245,* 172–178.

Magni, G., Moreschi, C., Rigatti-Luchini, S., & Merskey, H. (1994). Prospective study on the relationship between depressive symptoms and chronic musculoskeletal pain. *Pain, 56,* 289–297.

McBeth, J., Macfarlane, G., Benjamin, S., Morris, S., & Silman, A. (1999). The association between tender points, psychological distress, and adverse childhood experiences: A community-based study. *Arthritis & Rheumatism, 42,* 1397–1404.

McWilliams, L., Cox, B., & Enns, M. (2003). Mood and anxiety disorders associated with chronic pain: An examination in a nationally representative sample. *Pain, 106,* 127–133.

Meagher, M. W. (2004). Links between traumatic family violence and chronic pain: Biopsychosocial pathways and treatment implications. In K. A. Kendall-Tackett (Ed.), *Health consequences of abuse in the family: A clinical guide for evidence-based practice* (pp. 155–177). Washington, DC: American Psychological Association.

Meagher, M. W., Arnau, R. C., & Rhudy, J. L. (2001). Pain and emotion: Effects of affective picture modulation. *Psychosomatic Medicine, 63,* 79–90.

Molnar, B., Buka, S., & Kessler, R. (2001). Child sexual abuse and subsequent psychopathology: Results from the National Comorbidity Survey. *American Journal of Public Health, 91,* 753–760.

Monahan, K., & Forgash, C. (2000). Enhancing the health care experiences of adult female survivors of childhood sexual abuse. *Women's Health, 30*(4), 27–41.

Nichols, H. B., & Harlow, B. L. (2004). Childhood abuse and risk of smoking onset. *Journal of Epidemiology & Community Health, 58,* 402–406.

Petty, C., Sachs-Ericsson, N., & Joiner, T. (2004). Interpersonal dysfunction: Cause or result of depressive disorders. *Journal of Affective Disorders, 81*(2), 115–122.

Plant, E. A., & Sachs-Ericsson, N. (2004). Racial and ethnic differences in depression: The roles of social support and meeting basic needs. *Journal of Consulting and Clinical Psychology, 72,* 41–52.

Rende, R., & Plomin, R. (1992). Diathesis-stress models of psychopathology: A quantitative genetic perspective. *Applied & Preventive Psychology, 1*(4), 177–182.

Romans, S., Belaise, C., Martin, J., Morris, E., & Raffi, A. (2002). Childhood abuse and later medical disorders in women: An epidemiological study. *Psychotherapy & Psychosomatics, 71*(3), 141–150.

Romans, S., Martin, J., Anderson, J., O'Shea, M., & Mullen, P. (1995). Factors that mediate between child sexual abuse and adult psychological outcome. *Psychological Medicine, 25,* 127–142.

Roosa, M., Reinholtz, C., & Angelini, P. (1999). The relation of child sexual abuse and depression in young women: Comparisons across four ethnic groups. *Journal of Abnormal Child Psychology, 27*(1), 65–76.

Sachs-Ericsson, N., Blazer, D., Plant, E. A., & Arnow, B. (2005). Childhood sexual and physical abuse and the one-year prevalence of medical problems in the National Comorbidity Study. *Health Psychology, 24,* 32–40.

Sachs-Ericsson, N., Kendall-Tackett, K., & Hernandez, A. (2007). Childhood abuse, chronic pain and depression in the National Comorbidity Survey. *Child Abuse & Neglect, 3,* 531–547.

Sachs-Ericsson, N., Verona, E., Joiner, T., & Preacher, K. (2006). Parental verbal abuse and the mediating role of self-criticism in adult internalizing disorders. *Journal of Affective Disorders, 93*(1–3), 71–78.

Scarinci, I. C., McDonald-Haile, J., Bradley, L. A., & Richter, J. E. (1994). Altered pain perception and psychosocial features among women with gastrointestinal disorders and history of abuse: A preliminary model. *American Journal of Medicine, 97,* 108–118.

Schachter, C. L., Radomsky, N. A., Stalker, C. A., & Teram, E. (2004). Women survivors of child sexual abuse: How can health professionals promote healing? *Canadian Family Physician, 50,* 405–412.

Schnurr, P., & Green, B. L. (2004). Understanding relationships among trauma, post-traumatic stress disorder, and health outcomes. *Advances in Mind-Body Medicine, 20*(1), 18–29.

Schnurr, P. P., & Spiro, A. (1999). Combat exposure, posttraumatic stress disorder symptoms, and health behaviors as predictors of self-reported physical health in older veterans. *Journal of Nervous and Mental Disorders, 187,* 353–359.

Schoenbaum, M., Unutzer, J., Sherbourne, C., Duan, N., Rubenstein, L. V., Miranda, J., et al. (2001). Cost-effectiveness of practice-initiated quality improvement for depression: Results of a randomized controlled trial. *Journal of the American Medical Association, 286,* 1325–1330.

Shiffman, S. (1993). Assessing smoking patterns and motives. *Journal of Consulting and Clinical Psychology, 61,* 732–742.

Sidebotham, P., Golding, J., & the ALSPAC Study Team. (2001). Child maltreatment in the "children of the nineties": A longitudinal study of parental risk factors. *Child Abuse & Neglect, 25,* 1177–1200.

Springs, F. E., & Friedrich, W. N. (1992). Health risk behaviors and medical sequelae of childhood sexual abuse. *Mayo Clinic Proceedings, 67,* 527–532.

Stahl, S. (2002). Does depression hurt? *Journal of Clinical Psychiatry, 63,* 273–274.

Stein, M. B., & Barrett-Connor, E. (2000). Sexual assault and physical health: Findings from a population-based study of older adults. *Psychosomatic Medicine, 62,* 838–843.

Talley, N. J., Fett, S. L., & Zinsmeister, A. R. (1995). Self-reported abuse and gastrointestinal disease in outpatients: Association with irritable bowel-type symptoms. *American Journal of Gastroenterology, 90,* 366–371.

Thakkar, R., & McCanne, T. (2000). The effects of daily stressors on physical health in women with and without a childhood history of sexual abuse. *Child Abuse & Neglect, 24,* 209–221.

Thompson, M. P., Arias, I., Basile, K. C., & Desai, S. (2002). The association between childhood physical and sexual victimization and health problems in adulthood in a nationally representative sample of women. *Journal of Interpersonal Violence, 17,* 1115–1129.

Thompson, M. P., Kingree, J. B., & Desai, S. (2004). Gender differences in long-term health consequences of physical abuse of children: Data from a nationally representative survey. *American Journal of Public Health, 94,* 599–604.

Turner, H. A., & Muller, P. A. (2004). Long-term effects of child corporal punishment on depressive symptoms in young adults: Potential moderators and mediators. *Journal of Family Issues, 25,* 761–782.

Verona, E., & Sachs-Ericsson, N. (2005). The intergenerational transmission of externalizing behaviors in adult participants: The mediating role of childhood abuse. *Journal of Consulting and Clinical Psychology, 73,* 1135–1145.

Waldinger, R. J., Schulz, M. S., Barsky, A. J., & Ahern, D. K. (2006). Mapping the road from childhood trauma to adult somatization: The role of attachment. *Psychosomatic Medicine, 68,* 129–135.

Walker, E. A., Gelfand, A., Katon, J., Koss, M., Von Korff, M., Bernstein, D., et al. (1999). Adult health status of women with histories of childhood abuse. *American Journal of Medicine, 107,* 332–339.

Walsh, C. A., Jamieson, E., MacMillan, H., & Boyle, M. (2007). Child abuse and chronic pain in a community survey of women. *Journal of Interpersonal Violence, 22,* 1536–1554.

Williamson, D. F., Thompson, T. J., Anda, R. F., Dietz, W. H., & Felitti, V. (2002). Body weight and obesity in adults and self-reported abuse in childhood. *International Journal of Obesity, 26,* 1075–1082.

Wilson, A. E., Calhoun, K. S., & Bernat, J. A. (1999). Risk recognition and trauma-related symptoms among sexually revictimized women. *Journal of Consulting and Clinical Psychology, 67,* 705–710.

Yehuda, R., Boisoneau, D., Lowy, M. T., & Giller, E. L. (1995). Dose-response changes in plasma cortisol and lymphocyte glucocorticoid receptors following dexamethasone administration in combat veterans with and without posttraumatic stress disorder. *Archives of General Psychiatry, 52,* 583–593.

Zelman, D., Howland, E., Nichols, S., & Cleeland, C. (1991). The effects of induced mood on laboratory pain. *Pain, 46,* 105–111.

Zuravin, S. J., & Fontanella, C. (1999). The relationship between child sexual abuse and major depression among low-income women: A function of growing up experiences? *Child Maltreatment, 4*(1), 3–12.

Birth Trauma and Its Sequelae

CHERYL TATANO BECK, DNSc, CNM, FAAN

School of Nursing, University of Connecticut, Storrs, Connecticut, USA

Reported international rates of posttraumatic stress disorder due to birth trauma range as high as 5.9%. Trauma associated with perinatal events, however, is often lacking in discussions of women's trauma. The main focus of this article is on the description of 3 qualitative studies on birth trauma, posttraumatic stress disorder due to birth trauma, and the anniversary of a traumatic birth. Birth trauma is placed in the context of trauma theory. Implications for clinical practice are addressed.

An *extreme traumatic stressor* is defined in the *Diagnostic and Statistical Manual of Mental Disorders* (4th ed., text rev.; American Psychiatric Association, 2000) as

> involving direct personal experience of an event that involves actual or threatened death or serious injury, or other threat to one's physical integrity; or witnessing an event that involves death, injury, or a threat to the physical integrity of another person; or learning about unexpected or violent death, serious harm, or threat of death or injury experienced by a family member or other close associate. (p. 464)

Intense fear, horror, and helplessness are responses to this trauma. Three clusters of symptoms that result from experiencing trauma are (a) persistent reexperiencing of the trauma, (b) numbing and persistent avoidance of triggers related to the trauma, and (c) increased arousal. Examples of trauma that persons can directly experience include military combat, sexual assault, terrorist attack, natural disasters, and automobile accidents (American Psychiatric Association, 2000).

Kendall-Tackett (2005) identified three differences between women's and men's experiences of stress and trauma: (a) Women's stress and trauma are frequently relationally based, (b) women are more vulnerable to depression and perhaps posttraumatic stress disorder (PTSD), and (c) women are more vulnerable to physical illnesses that are stress related. Trauma related to pregnancy, birth, and the postpartum period (perinatal events) can occur in women and impact the rest of their lives (Smart, 2003). Kendall-Tackett brought attention to the fact that trauma associated with perinatal events is often lacking in discussions of women's trauma.

Birth trauma is defined as "an event occurring during the labor and delivery process that involves actual or threatened serious injury or death to the mother or her infant. The birthing woman experiences intense fear, helplessness, loss of control, and horror" (Beck, 2004a, p. 28). The terms *birth trauma* and *traumatic childbirth* are used interchangeably in this article, whose main focus is on the description of a series of qualitative studies on birth trauma, the anniversary of birth trauma, and PTSD due to that trauma. Dissociation and birth trauma are also discussed. The article ends with implications for clinical practice.

International rates of PTSD due to birth trauma range from 1.7% in Sweden (Wijma, Soderqiust, & Wijma, 1997) to 5.9% in Nigeria (Adewuya, Ologun, & Ibigbami, 2006). The rates of women who do not have a formal diagnosis of PTSD but experience some posttraumatic stress symptoms due to a traumatic childbirth are substantially higher, that is 34% of a U.S. sample (Soet, Brack, & Dilorio, 2003) and 21.4% of a Dutch sample (Olde et al., 2005).

In the past 10 years researchers have focused on identifying predictors of women who perceive their childbirth as being traumatic. These risk factors include a high level of obstetric intervention (Creedy, Shocket, & Horsfall, 2000), dissatisfaction with the care received during the delivery process (Cigoli, Gilli, & Saita, 2006), feelings of powerlessness during childbirth (Nicholls & Ayers, 2007), premature delivery (Holditch-Davis, Bartlett, Blickman, & Miles, 2003), a history of psychiatric problems (Adewuya et al., 2006), previous counseling related to childbirth (Soderquist, Wijma, & Wijma, 2006), anxiety in pregnancy (Zaers, Waschke, & Ehlert, 2008), and history of sexual abuse (Simkin & Klaus, 2004; Soet et al., 2003).

Long-term effects of PTSD due to birth trauma are coming to the forefront as research on the more chronic nature of trauma due to childbirth is being conducted. Some of these troubling effects include detrimental relationships with partners, sexual dysfunction, fear of childbirth, and difficulties with mother–infant relationships (Ayers, Eagle, & Waring, 2006; Nicholls & Ayers, 2007).

BIRTH TRAUMA: IN THE EYE OF THE BEHOLDER

The phrase "beauty is in the eye of the beholder" was first penned by Margaret Wolfe Hungerford in 1878 in her novel *Molly Bawn*. As Beck (2004a) discovered in her phenomenological study of 40 women, beauty is not the only quality or experience that lies in the eye of the beholder. A traumatic childbirth also does. In that study, 23 women from New Zealand, 8 from the United States, 6 from Australia, and 3 from the United Kingdom were recruited via the Internet, mainly through a charitable trust, Trauma and Birth Stress (TABS; www.tabs.org.nz). The mean age of the women was 34 years. Regarding parity, 24 women were multiparas, whereas 16 were primiparas. Of the women, 34 were married, 3 divorced, and 3 single. A total of 22 mothers had vaginal births, and 18 had Caesarean births. Fifteen of the 40 women reported their educational level. Only 2 of these 15 women did not have at least a college degree.

In this study, women were asked to describe their traumatic childbirth experiences. From Colaizzi's (1978) data analysis method for a phenomenological study, four themes emerged from the 40 stories the women had written. Together the following four themes described the essence of a traumatic childbirth:

> Theme 1. To care for me: Was that too much to ask?
> Theme 2. To communicate with me: Why was this neglected?
> Theme 3. To provide safe care: You betrayed my trust and I felt powerless.
> Theme 4. The end justifies the means: At whose expense? At what price?

Why was it that one woman could have had an emergency Caesarean birth or a postpartum hemorrhage and perceived that her labor and delivery was traumatic, whereas another woman would not perceive it as such a negative experience? These four themes helped provide an answer to this question (Beck, 2004a). By not feeling cared for; by feeling that nurses, midwives, or physicians had not communicated with them; by feeling powerless; and by perceiving that their own experiences did not matter to others, women felt systematically stripped of protective layers during such a vulnerable time as labor and delivery. Women used adjectives such as "cold" and "mechanical" to describe the care they received during the delivery process. Mothers shared that they felt alone, abandoned, and stripped of their dignity. As one mother painfully shared, "The labor care has hurt deep in my soul and I have no words to describe the hurt. I was treated like nothing, just someone to get data from" (Beck, 2004a, p. 32).

Women shared how, at times, they felt invisible as the labor and delivery staff spoke to one another as if the mother were not in the room. A woman who was having her first baby recalled the following:

> After an hour of trying to deliver the baby with a vacuum extractor, the obstetrician said it was too late for an emergency Caesarean. The baby was truly stuck. By now the doctors are acting like I'm not there. The attending physician was saying, "We may have lost this bloody baby." The hospital staff discussed my baby's possible death in front of me and argued in front of me just as if I weren't there. (Beck, 2004a, pp. 32–33)

"Loss of control" and "powerlessness" were words used by some women to describe their terror during labor and delivery as they feared for their lives and/or their unborn infants' lives. Having survived a traumatic birth, women often felt as if no one cared at all about what they had gone through. Family, friends, and clinicians all celebrated the outcome of the delivery process: a healthy infant. The mother's birth trauma was pushed into the background. The following quote vividly illustrates this:

> I was congratulated for how "quickly and easily" the baby came out and that he scored a perfect 10! The worst thing was that nobody acknowledged that I had a bad time. Everyone was so pleased it had gone so well! I felt as if I had been raped! (Beck, 2004a, p. 34)

The chronic nature of birth trauma is the focus of the following section, in which mothers' experiences of the anniversaries of their traumatic childbirths are revealed.

ANNIVERSARY REACTIONS

Anniversary reactions are emotionally charged episodes timed to a person's previously experienced trauma wherein the person has an increase in psychiatric and/or physical symptoms (Weiss, 1958). The increase in this distressing symptomatology is precipitated by triggers of the upcoming date of the traumatizing event. Anniversary reactions have been reported, for instance, in Gulf War veterans (Morgan, Hill, Fox, Kingham, & Southwick, 1999) and mental health disaster relief workers on the anniversary of the New York World Trade Center's "ground zero" on September 11 (Daly et al., 2008). Symptoms that individuals must contend with at anniversary time can include numbness, sleep disturbances, intrusive memories, irritability, and anger. Van der Kolk, McFarlane, and Weisaeth (1996) warned that anniversaries of trauma can be especially problematic for persons who develop PTSD. Anniversaries of trauma can reactivate symptoms associated with PTSD that had decreased over the previous year (e.g., the 9/11 first anniversary; Jordan, 2003).

Anniversary of Birth Trauma: Failure to Rescue

"Failure to rescue" was a phrase used by Beck (2006) to describe how not only health care providers but also family and friends failed to rescue and support women during the yearly anniversary of their traumatic births. The term "failure to rescue" was first used by Silber, Williams, Krakauer, and Schwartz (1992) to describe unnecessary deaths that occurred in hospitals as a complication of surgery. Beck broadened the use of this term to childbearing women because of the invisibility of the phenomenon of the anniversary of birth trauma. In this case, failure to rescue did not result in an unnecessary death but instead to the unnecessary suffering and decreased quality of life that women had to endure during the period of time surrounding the anniversary of their traumatic births.

Beck's (2006) phenomenological study on the anniversary of birth trauma involved 37 women who participated via the Internet. A recruitment notice was placed on the Web site of TABS, the charitable trust out of New Zealand. Mothers in the study represented the countries of the United States, New Zealand, Australia, the United Kingdom, and Canada. Of the women, 94% were married, 3% single, and 3% divorced. Moreover, 58% were primiparas, and 42% were multiparas. Regarding type of delivery, 58% of the sample had vaginal births, and 42% had Caesarean births. Of the 37 women, 29 reported their education: 19 of these 29 women held a college degree or higher degree. Mothers sent their descriptions of their experiences of the anniversaries of their traumatic births to the researcher via the Internet.

Just as with the birth trauma study, Beck (2006) used Colaizzi's (1978) method of data analysis. Four themes revealed the essence of mothers' anniversary experiences: (a) The prologue: An agonizing time; (b) The actual day: A celebration of a birthday or the torment of an anniversary; (c) The epilogue: A fragile state; and (d) Subsequent anniversaries: For better or worse.

It was not just the one day of the anniversary that women struggled through but also the time preceding and following the day. Mothers wrote about being plagued with distressing thoughts and emotions during the weeks and months prior to the anniversary day. The following quote is one such example:

> The entire 2 days before the anniversary I watch the clock and relive all
> the hell I know that a year or two or three now ago for the first 30 plus

> hours of labor I was hanging in there suffering but dealing with the pain
> virtually alone. (Beck, 2006, p. 384)

Women were affected not only emotionally but also physically by the anniversary that loomed near. For example, asthma or psoriasis flared up as flashbacks to the birth trauma increased.

Complicating the anniversary for women who had experienced birth trauma was the fact that the day was also their child's birthday, a supposedly joyous day and cause for celebration. The concept of time played an important but distressing role during the actual anniversary day. Women frequently shared how they relieved every moment of that fateful day synchronized to the clock.

Some women in the study could not celebrate their child's birthday on the actual day. A random day would be picked to hold the birthday party, as is illustrated by this quote:

> We made a cake on a random day. I never told my son it was coming
> up. I brought him things and wrapped them but he doesn't know what
> they are for. I kissed him and told him before I went to work Happy
> Birthday but only when he was asleep. (Beck, 2006, p. 387)

Another strategy women used to survive the actual day of the anniversary was to physically get away, and so vacations were planned. Women did whatever they needed to do to protect themselves and to prevent the actual birthday from triggering the traumatic memories.

During the post-anniversary period, women were in a fragile state. Surviving the actual day that commemorated their traumatic childbirth took a huge toll on mothers. Time to recuperate was needed so that they could heal from the reopening of their emotional wounds. As this woman powerfully shared,

> As hard as I try to move away from the trauma, at birthday anniversary
> time I am pulled straight back as if on a giant rubber band into the midst
> of it all and spend MONTHS AFTER trying to pull myself away from it
> again. (Beck, 2006, p. 387, emphasis in the original)

No clear pattern emerged in Beck's (2006) study regarding women who had experienced more than one anniversary. For some mothers, each anniversary got a little bit easier to cope with, but for other women, the experience did not improve. The following excerpt from a mother who was about to celebrate her child's fourth birthday illustrates this:

> His birthday sits as a permanent barrier both in my relationship with my
> husband and my sense of attachment to my child. Although this is getting

better year by year, I am not sure it will every really disappear. The reawakening of the birth each birthday does mean I think again about what happened, my role in it, what I would have done to prevent it from happening and my sadness at what was taken away from me. The decisions I made that led down the path to the birth trauma haunt me. (Beck, 2006, pp. 387–388)

As stated earlier, up to approximately 6% of women suffer from PTSD secondary to birth trauma. What is it like for mothers to experience this anxiety disorder while trying to care for their newborn infants? The next section answers this question.

PTSD DUE TO CHILDBIRTH: THE AFTERMATH

In Beck's (2004b) third qualitative study via the Internet she investigated the experiences of PTSD due to birth trauma among 38 mothers. Just as in her previous studies women were recruited by a notice placed on the TABS Web site. In this study, 22 women were from New Zealand, 7 from the United States, 6 from Australia, and 3 from the United Kingdom. The majority of the sample was married (90%), was multiparas (68%), and had had vaginal births (55%). Of the 38 women, 17 shared their level of education. Only 3 of the 17 women reported having less than a college degree.

In the phenomenological study, women sent their stories to the researcher via the Internet. The TABS charitable trust was again instrumental in the recruitment of women across the globe. Mothers' stories of their experiences of PTSD due to birth trauma were analyzed using Colaizzi's (1978) method. Five themes described the essence of PTSD due to childbirth (see Figure 1).

Theme 1. Going to the Movies: Please Don't Make Me Go!

Flashbacks and nightmares of the traumatic birth haunted women. Mothers used the image of a mental videotape of their birth trauma running on automatic replay. Women felt as if there were loop tracks imprinted in their brains. One woman, who had failed a vacuum extraction that was then followed by a forceps delivery and fourth-degree laceration, disclosed the following:

I lived in two worlds, the videotape of the birth and the "real" world. The videotape felt more real. I lived in my own bubble, not quite connecting with anyone. I could hear and communicate, but experienced interaction with others as a spectator. The "videotape" ran constantly for 4 months. (Beck, 2004b, p. 219)

Theme		Theme
1	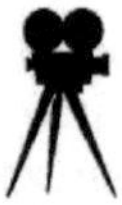	Going to the movies: Please don't make me go!
2	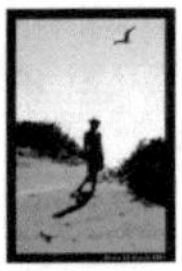	A shadow of myself: Too numb to try to change
3	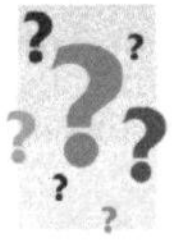	Seeking to have questions answered and wanting to talk, talk, talk
4	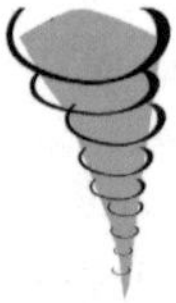	The dangerous trio of anger, anxiety, and depression: Spiraling downward
5	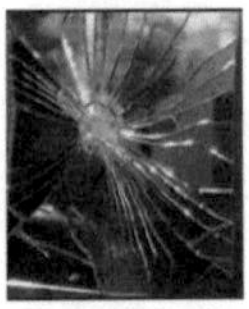	Isolation from the world of motherhood: Dreams shattered

FIGURE 1 Five essential themes of posttraumatic stress disorder due to childbirth. From "Post-Traumatic Stress Disorder Due to Childbirth: The Aftermath," by C. T. Beck, 2004, *Nursing Research, 53,* p. 220. Reprinted with permission of Lippincott Williams & Wilkins.

Theme 2. A Shadow of Myself: Too Numb to Try to Change

Women described feeling numb, like an empty shell, detached, and at times actually dissociating, as this mother who had an emergency Caesarean birth and postpartum hemorrhage explained:

> I had a drip, a catheter, and was silent. I felt completely numb. I did what was required and I felt my head was floating way above my body. I struggled to bring it back onto my shoulders. I still feel dissociated like this sometimes. (Beck, 2004b, p. 220)

Theme 3. Seeking to Have Questions Answered and Wanting to Talk, Talk, Talk

Mothers became obsessed at times trying to understand and to make sense of what had gone so wrong with their labors and deliveries. Family, friends, and clinicians became tired and impatient listening to the women talking excessively about their birth trauma. This mother of twins remembered that she

> was so devastated at the people's lack of empathy. I told myself what a bad person I was for needing to talk. I felt like the Ancient Mariner doomed to forever be plucking at people's sleeves and trying to tell them my story which they didn't want to hear. (Beck, 2004b, p. 221)

Theme 4. The Dangerous Trio of Anger, Anxiety, and Depression: Spiraling Downward

When suffering from PTSD due to childbirth, women experienced emotions at an exaggerated level. Anger became rage, anxiety spiraled into panic attacks, and at times depression led mothers to contemplate suicide. A glimpse into this anger is provided by the words of this mother:

> Powerful seething anger would overwhelm me without warning. To manage it I would go still and quiet, then eventually "come to," realizing that one or all of the children were crying and I had no idea for how long. (Beck, 2004b, p. 221)

Theme 5. Isolation from the World of Motherhood: Dreams Shattered

As with all PTSD, the person tries to avoid any triggers of the original trauma. Some mothers grappling with PTSD secondary to childbirth tried to distance themselves from their infants and separated themselves from other mothers and babies. Detrimental implications can be envisioned for the developing mother–infant relationship. As one mother painfully shared,

> My child turned 3 years old a few weeks ago. I suppose the pain was not so acute this time. I actually made him a birthday cake and was grateful that I could go to work and not think about the significance of the day. The pain was less, but it was replaced by a numbness that still worries me. I hope that as time passes I can forge some kind of real closeness with this child. I am still unable to tell him I love him, but I can now hold him and have times when I am proud of him. I have come a long, long way. (Beck, 2004b, p. 222)

DISSOCIATION AND BIRTH TRAUMA

Dissociation during a traumatic labor and delivery has been reported. In a longitudinal study of 248 women in The Netherlands, van Son, Verkerk, van der Hart, Komprae, and Pop (2005) found that 19% of the women experienced high perinatal dissociation. The Peritraumatic Dissociative Experiences Questionnaire (Marmar, Weiss, & Metzler, 1997) was used to assess dissociation during childbirth. This is a 10-item self-report instrument assessing such experiences as derealization, disorientation, amnesia, altered time perception, and out-of-body experience. The reported alpha correlation was $r = .81$.

Peritraumatic dissociation occurred in 70% of 118 women in The Netherlands who had experienced pregnancy loss (Engelhard, van den Hout, Kindt, Arntz, & Schouten, 2003). For pregnant women with abuse histories, labor and delivery may trigger flashbacks from the original trauma and lead to using dissociation as a coping mechanism (Cole, Scoville, & Flynn, 1996).

In a case study of an adult survivor of childhood sexual abuse and her childbearing and breastfeeding experiences (Beck, in press), this mother vividly described how during her labor and delivery she dissociated:

> A haze of hospital labor room, nakedness, vulnerability, pain. Silence, stretching, breathing, pain, terror, and then I found myself 7 years old again, and sitting outside my parents' house in the car of a family acquaintance, being digitally raped. The flashback to the abuse that I had experienced 23 years ago was not new. I always knew it had happened. What was different this time was that I felt the emotional response to it. I had never felt that before. In the midst of transition of the birth of my first baby, I finally felt it all in one shocking moment: the anguish, the shame, the horror, the violation, the massive breach of trust, the grief, the betrayal, the confusion, the despair and the dirtiness. I felt like I had left my body. I know now that I had dissociated. But all I knew then was that I wasn't there with my body, my baby any more. Of course, my body was still there. Noises from the room were muffled and muted. Faraway voices of my mother and the midwife remarked upon how composed I was. How good I was being. How little noise I was making.

IMPLICATIONS FOR CLINICAL PRACTICE

The fact that some of the women in Beck's (2004a, 2004b, 2006) studies were still struggling 3 to 4 years after their traumatic birth indicates ongoing mental health issues that have not been resolved. It is not known if women in these three qualitative studies had mental health problems prior to birth. A few mothers did volunteer that they had experienced prior trauma, such as rape and/or childhood sexual abuse. More research needs to be focused on prior mental health issues of women before childbirth.

Alder, Stadlmayr, Tschudin, and Bitzer (2006) have developed a multi-level counseling approach that includes counseling during the postpartum period and also during a subsequent pregnancy. The first possibility to assess for a negative birth experience comes while the mother is still in the hospital. Alder and colleagues suggested questions that can be used to assess the birth experience in the postpartum period. These questions focus on four domains: overall birth experience, pain, care received during labor and delivery, and obstetric procedures. When a woman returns to her obstetrical care provider around 6 weeks after delivery, this routine visit presents a second possible time to inquire about posttraumatic stress symptoms. At either of these times, mothers can be screened for posttraumatic stress symptoms. Alder et al. provided suggested questions to assess avoidance, intrusion, and arousal.

Based on her literature review, Ayers (2004) developed a model of vulnerability and risk factors for postpartum PTSD (see Figure 2). By screening for these predictors clinicians can use this model for primary prevention

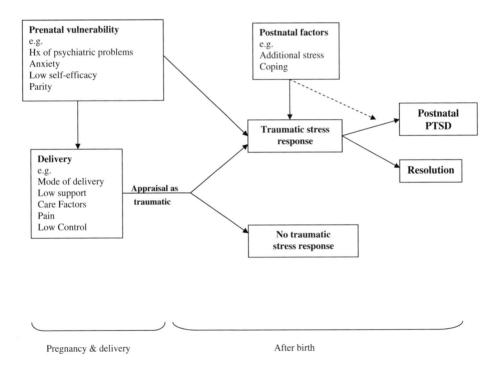

FIGURE 2 Model of vulnerability and risk factors for postpartum posttraumatic stress disorder (PTSD). Hx = history. From "Delivery as a Traumatic Event: Prevalence, Risk Factors, and Treatment for Postnatal Posttraumatic Stress Disorder," by S. Ayers, 2004, *Clinical Obstetrics and Gynecology, 47,* p. 562. Reprinted with permission of Lippincott Williams & Wilkins.

by identifying vulnerable women while they are still pregnant. Ayers suggested that these high-risk women can be offered alternative birthing options. Also, their charts can be marked so that labor and delivery staff can provide extra support to them during labor.

Just as new mothers are now being screened for postpartum depression after delivery, so do women need to be screened for posttraumatic stress symptoms related to delivery. The Modified Perinatal Post-Traumatic Stress Disorder Questionnaire (Modified PPQ) is an example of an instrument currently available that has been developed specifically for assessing PTSD symptoms related to childbirth (Callahan, Borja, & Hynan, 2006). The Modified PPQ consists of 14 items assessing posttraumatic stress symptoms related to childbirth. Items measure persistent reexperiencing of intrusiveness, avoidance, and hyperarousal symptoms, which are the three criteria used in the *Diagnostic and Statistical Manual of Mental Disorders* (4th ed., text rev.) for diagnosing PTSD (American Psychiatric Association, 2000). Response options are on a 5-point Likert scale from 0 = *not at all* to 4 = *often, for more than a month*. The total possible score on the Modified PPQ can range from 0 to 56. The PPQ was originally developed as a dichotomous scale (DeMier, Hynan, Harris, & Manniello, 1996) but was modified to enhance clinical utility.

Callahan et al. (2006) assessed the psychometrics of the Modified PPQ using an Internet-based survey completed by 179 women. Of this sample, 47 mothers had had premature infants, 11 had had medically fragile infants, and 86 had had healthy full-term infants. Internal consistency of the total Modified PPQ was r = .90. Factor analysis revealed that the instrument was composed of three components. The largest component of the Modified PPQ accounted for 44% of the total variance in scores and consisted of items related to hyperarousal. The internal consistency of this component was r = .86. The next largest component accounted for 13% of the total score variance and had an internal consistency reliability of r = .80. This component reflected items in avoidance. The third component, reflecting persistent reexperiencing, accounted for 7% of the variance and had a lower alpha of r = .66. Callahan and colleagues (2006) recommended a cutoff score of 19 or above, which yielded a sensitivity of 0.82 for correctly identifying mothers in need of mental health referral.

An example of another instrument available to screen for clinical PTSD is the PTSD Symptom Scale (Foa, Riggs, Dancu, & Rothbaum, 1993). The PTSD Symptom Scale has been adapted into the Posttraumatic Diagnostic Scale (Foa, 1995). Another scale that has been used with postpartum samples is the Traumatic Event Scale (Wijma et al., 1997). Instruments for screening women for posttraumatic stress symptoms are now being assessed for their psychometrics. What is also needed is research on counseling strategies for women with posttraumatic stress symptoms due to childbirth.

In conclusion, it is important that birth trauma and its resulting PTSD be recognized by clinicians. Screening needs to be done routinely because the secondary effects of women's suffering from PTSD can affect their infants, their other children, and their entire families. Counselors need to be proactive in preparing women who have experienced birth trauma for the yearly anniversary of their child's birth. Anniversary effects need to be addressed preventively (Jordan, 2003).

REFERENCES

Adewuya, A. O., Ologun, Y. A., & Ibigbami, O. S. (2006). Post-traumatic stress disorder after childbirth in Nigerian women: Prevalence and risk factors. *BJOG: An International Journal of Obstetrics and Gynecology, 113*, 284–288.

Alder, J., Stadlmayr, W., Tschudin, S., & Bitzer, J. (2006). Post-traumatic symptoms after childbirth: What should we offer? *Journal of Psychosomatic Obstetrics & Gynecology, 27*, 107–112.

American Psychiatric Association. (2000). *Diagnostic and statistical manual of mental disorders* (4th ed., text rev.). Washington, DC: Author.

Ayers, S. (2004). Delivery as a traumatic event: Prevalence, risk factors, and treatment for postnatal posttraumatic stress disorder. *Clinical Obstetrics and Gynecology, 47*, 552–567.

Ayers, S., Eagle, A., & Waring, H. (2006). The effects of childbirth-related post-traumatic stress disorder on women and their relationships: A qualitative study. *Psychology, Health & Medicine, 11*, 389–398.

Beck, C. T. (in press). Adult survivor of child sexual abuse and her breastfeeding experience: A case study. *MCN: The American Journal of Maternal Child Nursing.*

Beck, C. T. (2004a). Birth trauma: In the eye of the beholder. *Nursing Research, 53*, 28–35.

Beck, C. T. (2004b). Post-traumatic stress disorder due to childbirth: The aftermath. *Nursing Research, 53*, 216–224.

Beck, C. T. (2006). The anniversary of birth trauma: Failure to rescue. *Nursing Research, 55*, 381–390.

Callahan, J. L., Borja, S. E., & Hynan, M. T. (2006). Modification of the Perinatal PTSD Questionnaire to enhance clinical utility. *Journal of Perinatology, 26*, 533–539.

Cigoli, V., Gilli, G., & Saita, E. (2006). Relational factors in psychopathological responses to childbirth. *Journal of Psychosomatic Obstetrics and Gynecology, 27*, 91–97.

Colaizzi, P. F. (1978). Psychological research as the phenomenologist views it. In R. Valle & M. King (Eds.), *Existential phenomenological alternatives for psychology* (pp. 48–71). New York: Oxford University Press.

Cole, B. V., Scoville, M., & Flynn, L. T. (1996). Psychiatric advance practice nurses collaborative with certified nurse midwives in providing healthcare for pregnant women with histories of abuse. *Archives of Psychiatric Nursing, 10*, 229–234.

Creedy, D. K., Shocket, I. M., & Horsfall, J. (2000). Childbirth and the development of acute trauma symptoms: Incidence and contributing factors. *Birth, 27*, 104–111.

Daly, E. S., Gulliver, S. B., Zimering, R. T., Knight, J., Kamholz, B. W., & Nirussettem, S. B. (2008). Disaster mental health workers responding to ground zero: One year later. *Journal of Traumatic Stress, 21*, 227–230.

DeMier, R. L., Hynan, M. T., Harris, H. B., & Manniello, R. L. (1996). Perinatal stressors as predictors of symptoms of posttraumatic stress in mothers of infants at high risk. *Journal of Perinatology, 16,* 276–280.

Engelhard, I. M., van den Hout, M. A., Kindt, M., Arntz, A., & Schouten, E. (2003). Peritraumatic dissociation and posttraumatic stress after pregnancy loss: A prospective study. *Behavior Research and Therapy, 41,* 67–78.

Foa, E. B. (1995). *The Posttraumatic Diagnostic Scale (PDS).* Minneapolis, MN: National Computer Systems.

Foa, E. B., Riggs, D. S., Dancu, C. V., & Rothbaum, B. (1993). Reliability and validity of a brief instrument for assessing post-traumatic stress disorder. *Journal of Trauma and Stress, 6,* 459–473.

Holditch-Davis, D., Bartlett, T. R., Blickman, A. L., & Miles, M. S. (2003). Posttraumatic stress symptoms in mothers of premature infants. *Journal of Obstetric, Gynecologic, & Neonatal Nursing, 32,* 161–171.

Hungerford, M. W. (1878). *Molly Bawn.* London: Smith, Elder.

Jordan, K. (2003). What we learned from the 9/11 first anniversary. *The Family Journal: Counseling and Therapy for Couples and Families, 11,* 110–116.

Kendall-Tackett, K. A. (2005). *Handbook of women, stress, and trauma.* New York: Brunner-Routledge.

Marmar, C. R., Weiss, D. S., & Metzler, T. J. (1997). The Peritraumatic Dissociative Experiences Questionnaire. In J. P. Wilson & T. M. Keane (Eds.), *Assessing psychological trauma and posttraumatic stress disorder* (pp. 412–428). New York: Guilford Press.

Morgan, C. A., Hill, S., Fox, P., Kingham, P., & Southwick, S. M. (1999). Anniversary reactions in Gulf War veterans: A follow up inquiry 6 years later after the war. *American Journal of Psychiatry, 156,* 1075–1079.

Nicholls, K., & Ayers, S. (2007). Childbirth related post-traumatic stress disorder in couples: A qualitative study. *British Journal of Health Psychology, 12,* 491–509.

Olde, E., van der Hart, O., Kleber, R. J., van Son, M. J. M., Wijnen, H. A. A., & Pop, V. J. M. (2005). Posttraumatic dissociation and emotions as predictors of PTSD symptoms following childbirth. *Journal of Trauma & Dissociation, 6,* 125–142.

Silber, J. H., Williams, S. V., Krakauer, H., & Schwartz, J. S. (1992). Hospital and patient failure to rescue. *Medical Care, 30,* 615–629.

Simkin, P., & Klaus, P. (2004). *When survivors give birth: Understanding and healing the effects of early sexual abuse on childbearing women.* Seattle, WA: Classic Day.

Smart, L. S. (2003). Old losses: A retrospective study of miscarriage and infant death 1926-1955. *Journal of Women and Aging, 15,* 71–91.

Soderquist, J., Wijma, B., & Wijma, K. (2006). The longitudinal course of post-traumatic stress after childbirth. *Journal of Psychosomatic Obstetrics and Gynecology, 27,* 113–119.

Soet, J. E., Brack, G. A., & Dilorio, C. (2003). Prevalence and predictors of women's experiences of psychological trauma during childbirth, *Birth, 30,* 36–46.

Van der Kolk, B. A., McFarlane, A. C., & Weisaeth, L. (1996). *Traumatic stress: The effects of overwhelming experience on mind, body, and soul.* New York: Guilford Press.

van Son, M., Verkerk, G., van der Hart, O., Komprae, I., & Pop, V. (2005). Prenatal depression, mode of delivery and perinatal dissociation as predictors of post-partum post-traumatic stress: An empirical study. *Clinical Psychology and Psychotherapy, 12,* 297–312.

Weiss, E. (1958). The clinical significance of the anniversary reaction. *General Practitioner, 27,* 117–119.

Wijma, K., Soderquist, J., & Wijma, B. (1997). Posttraumatic stress disorder after childbirth: A cross sectional study. *Journal of Anxiety Disorders, 11,* 587–597.

Zaers, S., Waschke, M., & Ehlert, U. (2008). Depressive symptoms and symptoms of post-traumatic stress disorder in women after childbirth. *Journal of Psychosomatic Obstetrics & Gynecology, 29,* 61–71.

"That Part of the Body is Just Gone": Understanding and Responding to Dissociation and Physical Health

TERRI J. HAVEN, MSW

Private Practice, West Springfield, Massachusetts, USA

The past 2 decades have brought a significant surge in interest and research regarding the ways in which psychological trauma relates to the physical body. Researchers now understand a great deal about how the brain and the body process traumatic experiences, as well as the increased likelihood of an array of physical health consequences associated with both childhood and adult trauma and posttraumatic stress disorder. Experts are increasingly challenging mind–body dualism through solid theoretical and clinical bases for the central importance of listening to and communicating with trauma clients' bodies as part of reducing the suffering and long-lasting consequences of trauma. This article integrates this growing body of knowledge through a particular focus on trauma-induced dissociation and the implications of the physical and neurological processes and consequences of dissociation on clients' ability to participate in caring for their own bodies. The author utilizes an in-depth clinical example of expanding relational trauma psychotherapy to include a focus on working directly with trauma-related sensorimotor and physiological sensations and patterns.

John[1] and I first met 3 years after he was violently and randomly attacked outside his home while walking to the store for cigarettes. He suffered severe injuries to his torso and was left with debilitating physical and psychological scars. Unfortunately, for those 3 years after the attack, John had received very little professional psychological support and had relied on psychiatric medications and his primary coping strategy of dissociation to survive. When we first met he sat very rigidly with his arms by his side, basically moved only his eyes, blinked frequently, and spoke in very short sentences.

When I asked about John's reasons for coming to therapy, he replied, "I don't know what else to do; they won't give me my meds if I don't come and you're the only person who would see me." In response to my inquiry about how life was different since the attack, John said, "My chest and back are just gone" and "I can't do anything or go anywhere anymore." Throughout this article, I invite you into several crucial parts of my evolving psychotherapy process with John to consider both the psychological and physical consequences of dissociation for complex trauma survivors.

TRAUMA AND THE BODY

There has been a tremendous surge in interest and research over the past two decades regarding the ways that psychological trauma relates to the body. Van der Kolk's (1994) seminal article, "The Body Keeps the Score," first signaled a shift in attention from a primary focus on the psychological to the neurobiological and the body in traumatic stress. Since then there have been enormous strides in how the brain and the body process traumatic experiences (see Van der Kolk, 2006, for a current, in-depth review of the clinical implications of neuroscience research). The physical health effects of traumatic events and experiences are also now receiving increasing research attention in the medical literature. For example, in the classic Adverse Childhood Experiences Study, Felitti and colleagues (1998) found that childhood trauma was associated with increased likelihood of adult cancer, ischemic heart disease, chronic lung problems, and other conditions that had no known or direct etiological basis in the childhood events. Allen (2001) recommended conceptualizing posttraumatic stress disorder as a chronic physical illness, using diabetes as a paradigm and providing education about self-care as a foundation. In addition to bringing together an array of meaningful contributions in the field of trauma and health, Schnurr and Green (2004), in a recent edited volume, proposed a model that explains the association of traumatic events and poor physical health through psychological, biological, attentional, and behavioral mechanisms and stressed the importance of an integrated approach to care.

The dualism of mind and body also continues to be challenged with major contributions such as *Waking the Tiger* (Levine, 1997), *Splintered Reflections* (Goodwin & Attias, 1999), *The Body Remembers* (Rothschild, 2000), *The Body Bears the Burden* (Scaer, 2001, 2007), *The Trauma Spectrum: Hidden Wounds and Human Resiliency* (Scaer, 2005), and *Trauma and the Body: A Sensorimotor Approach to Psychotherapy* (Ogden, Minton, & Pain, 2006). All of these authors, while traveling very similar paths albeit with slightly different focuses, present solid theoretical and clinical bases for the central importance of listening to and communicating with trauma clients' bodies as part of reducing the suffering and long-lasting consequences of trauma.

In previous work (Haven, 2002; Haven & Pearlman, 2004), I considered the importance of including attention to clients' bodies, particularly their physical health, within relational trauma psychotherapy and the role of dissociation in impacting both clients' and therapists' awareness and discussion of physical health. In building on that work, this article focuses not only on the consequences of dissociation of mental functions, but in particular on the physical and neurological processes and consequences of dissociation on clients' ability to participate in caring for their own bodies.

DEFINING AND UNDERSTANDING DISSOCIATION

The field has made tremendous strides and yet continues to face several challenges in efforts to further operationalize the working definitions of trauma-induced dissociation. Most recently, DePrince and Freyd (2007) provided an excellent in-depth discussion of the varying dimensions and considerations over the past two decades, the current state of the art, and the challenges for the future in regard to the evolving definitions and understanding of dissociation. DePrince and Freyd suggested that a dialectical view of dissociation may help resolve issues of the adaptive–maladaptive nature of dissociation: "Dissociation may be both a creative adaptation to an environmental insult that threatens survival . . . and a deficit that causes problems in other domains of life . . . that invokes the importance of examining context" (p. 139). These authors stressed the importance of continued work to "examine differences in pathological versus nonpathological views of dissociation . . . to not exclude relevant phenomena . . . to untangle the complicated picture of comorbidity between dissociation and other forms of trauma-related distress" (pp. 146–147).

My central understanding of dissociation has been informed by a relational trauma framework, in particular constructivist self-development theory (for detailed discussions of constructivist self-development theory, see McCann & Pearlman, 1990; Pearlman & Saakvitne, 1995; Saakvitne, Gamble, Pearlman, & Lev, 2000). Increasingly as I have come to expand the psychotherapy process related to dissociation to include the body, the context of freezing and tonic immobility (Allen, 2001; Foa, Zinbarg, & Rothbaum, 1992; Levine, 1997; Nijenhuis, Vanderlinden, & Spinhoven, 1998; Ogden, Minton et al., 2006) and the neurological functions of the brain in imprinting and processing trauma (Ogden, Minton et al., 2006; Van der Kolk, 2006; Wylie, 2004) have also become invaluable.

Constructivist self-development theory understands dissociation within the context of self-capacities or inner abilities to regulate internal psychological processes and experiences. (See Pearlman, 1998, for an in-depth discussion of self-capacities.) These capacities include the ability to regulate affect, maintain a sense of positive self-worth, and maintain an inner sense of connection to benign others; they are developed in the earliest relationships with central caregivers or attachment figures. When those important others are not attuned to the child, are physically or emotionally absent, or are abusive, the child's self-capacities are not adequately developed (Haven & Pearlman, 2004).

In adulthood, individuals with inadequately developed self-capacities struggle to tolerate or modulate their feelings. An often familiar solution to this struggle for many survivors is *dissociation*, a response to potential or experienced danger that disconnects feelings, whether the source is internal or external. Pearlman and Saakvitne (1995) explained the central importance of understanding dissociation both as an intrapsychic defense and, in psychotherapy, as an interpersonal process:

> Phenomenologically, it is the separation of mental systems that would ordinarily be integrated. It represents the severing of connections among mental contents and categories that would otherwise elaborate and augment one another. Theoretically, it provides the therapist an invaluable framework for understanding a range of intrapsychic and interpersonal occurrences in psychotherapy with trauma survivors. (p. 120)

Pearlman and Saakvitne continued (further referenced and applied by Haven & Pearlman in 2004) by defining the intrapsychic functions of dissociation as follows: (a) to separate oneself from intolerable affects, reflecting the *need not to feel*; (b) to separate oneself from traumatic memories and knowledge, reflecting the *need not to know*; (c) to separate from unacceptable aspects of oneself, reflecting the *need not to be oneself*; and (d) to separate from the interpersonal relationship, reflecting the *need to manage the threat that connection poses*.

John's use of dissociation as understood through this lens first came to light very early in our work together. He had been denied disability, had no means of income, and needed my assistance quickly to complete the necessary appeal paperwork. Completing the disability forms also was the first way that we discussed or even acknowledged John's body, as the questions required very detailed information in terms of his history, his daily activities, and his physical abilities/limitations. It was also primarily the only way John participated verbally in our early sessions.

Therapist: John, what does it feel like for us to be filling out these forms together? I'm aware that we're discussing some very private parts of your life before we really have a chance to get to know each other.

John: It doesn't really feel like anything. It's just there and needs to be done . . . that part of the body is just gone since it all happened anyway.

Therapist: John, what do you mean "gone"?

John: Haven't seen it and don't talk or think about it—just want to answer the questions they have to know, okay?

Therapist: Of course, John. Maybe another time we can try to understand more about part of your body being gone and not feeling like anything— would that be okay?

John: Maybe, but it won't do any good. You're really saving me though by doing this paperwork.

John needed *not to feel* the intensity of emotions related to his trauma, *not to know* the consequences for his body, and *to manage our relationship* through a fragmented focus on "idealizing" me as his savior. As that session came to an end:

Therapist: John, as we've worked on this application today I've noticed that your breathing became more shallow. This process is complicated, isn't it?

John: Yep. Kind of nervous.

Many trauma therapists have come to understand that dissociation is "contagious"; when a client is unaware of something, it is often difficult for the therapist to bring it to mind or keep it in his or her own awareness (Davies & Frawley, 1994; Haven, 2002; Haven & Pearlman, 2004; Pearlman & Saakvitne, 1995; Saakvitne et al., 2000). In that session with John, I was aware of feeling an unusual amount of anxiety within myself as he and I made our way through the questions on the application. I understood myself to be holding much of John's affect and therefore focused on broadening his awareness of his change in breathing in my efforts to help reduce his "nervousness." I didn't "remember" that his lungs had been seriously injured in the attack and that he used smoking cigarettes as a way to self-medicate and manage stress. I *needed not to know* about the horrible things that had been done to John's body or to consider the ways his body might still be impacted in the present moment.

THE EARLY PROCESS

For about the first year John and I saw each other weekly. He was unable to drive and depended initially on his elderly mother for transportation. His sense of terror and shame coupled with his mother's health issues limited John's ability to travel outside his home other than for medical appointments or to obtain basic necessities. Much of that first year our process focused on safety and stabilization, with a great deal of psychoeducation and the evolving development of a positive attachment within the therapeutic relationship. Gradually, John began to speak a little more, particularly as I showed gentle but consistent interest in and modeling of his safety and self-care and as we were successful in our appeal for disability benefits and subsequently adding an outreach support worker to our provider team.

Several months into therapy John began to have severe cuts across his hands and arms. In exploring these injuries with John, I learned that he was diligently trying to "save" a stray cat that had taken up residence outside his apartment and that he was letting the cat "play" roughly by attacking his hands and arms as his way of "showing the poor thing that he can trust me . . . he doesn't have anybody else." John became very focused on taking care of the cat (now named Star) and talking with me about the importance of taking the process with Star very slowly and "never giving up even if he takes a long time to trust coming inside." John initially had no conscious connection to any physical pain related to the cuts from such rough play with Star. However, over time he responded well to my concern for balancing his safety while supporting his goal of gaining Star's trust and eventually purchased thick gloves to protect his hands until Star stopped using his claws in that way. John's relationship with Star became a central metaphor for our work together, and eventually the "safety nets" we developed related to his relationship with Star were able to be applied more directly to John's overall sense of safety, self-care, self-worth, and connection with his body.

FROM THE INTRAPSYCHIC TO THE PHYSICAL: FIGHT, FLEE, OR FREEZE?

As John and I continued to work together, I was increasingly struck by his repeated experiences of himself as unable to fight or flee and instead remaining frozen in actions, words, and bodily movements. Sitting with John did indeed on occasion bring to mind the phrase of a "deer in headlights." I understood that by definition a person who is traumatized has experienced an inescapable sense of inability to either fight or flee. However, only through deeper understanding of the growing trauma-related literature related to the limitations of the fight-or-flight response, animal defense, freezing, and tonic immobility (Allen, 2001; Foa et al., 1992; Levine, 1997; Nijenhuis, Vanderlinden et al., 1998; Perry, Pollard, Blakley, Baker, & Vigilante, 1995) did I begin to have a more useful context for understanding this particular presentation of John's dissociation (and his strong identification with the terrified and traumatized cat that eventually became his companion and roommate).

Peter Levine (1997) developed an approach to trauma treatment called *somatic experiencing* that focuses on the belief that trauma is "locked" in the body and must be healed by accessing it in the body. Levine believes that all animals, including humans, are physically programmed by evolution to flee, fight, or freeze in the face of overwhelming threats to life. He notes that in humans, however, when these natural responses to danger are thwarted and people are helpless to prevent their own rape, or beating, or car accident, the unfinished defensive actions become blocked as undischarged energy in the nervous system. People remain physiologically frozen in an unfinished state of high biological readiness to react to the traumatic event, even long after the event has passed. Levine describes trauma victims as having been totally helpless and unable to move—physically and psychologically—and stresses that they must regain in therapy that lost capacity to move, to fight back, to live fully in their bodies as much as in their minds.

In reviewing the limitations of the fight-or-flight response, Nijenhuis, Vanderlinden et al. (1998) cited evidence that only a minority of women report having actively resisted sexual and physical abuse or rape, inasmuch as they perceived action to be useless or dangerous. Instead, passive defenses such as freezing, paralysis, and retreating into fantasy predominate. These authors also found that clients with dissociative disorders often display three behaviors akin to freezing in animals, namely analgesia, anesthesia, and behavioral immobility (Nijenhuis, Spinhoven, Vanderlinden, van Dyck, & van der Hart, 1998). Misslin (2003, p. 58) described freezing as "alert immobility," where there is complete cessation of movement except for respiration and movement of the eyes (much like John's initial presentation in therapy).

Ogden, Pain, and Fisher (2006) noted that "these incomplete actions of defense may subsequently manifest as chronic symptoms" (p. 272). These authors continued by noting that "individuals may experience their fight and flight muscles held in a chronically tightened patterns, have heightened and unstable aggressive impulses, or have a chronic lack of tone or sensation in a particular muscle group" (p. 272). In considering these concepts of freezing and dissociation, Allen (2001) noted that "although the parallels between freezing and dissociation seem compelling, there is a crucial difference between them . . . . dissociation entails disengaging from environmental stimuli . . . yet, the frozen animal is hypervigilant . . . freezing is a highly engaged, not detached, state" (p. 172). Allen continued by referencing Perry and colleagues' (1995) continuum of dissociative responses ranging from freezing to surrender, with surrender being consistent with tonic immobility, and emphasized the crucial focus on surrender as a better prototype for this aspect of dissociation.

At a point about a year and a half into our work and soon after we had increased sessions to twice a week, John and I spoke directly about the evening he was attacked. His description aptly reflected a movement from a very hypervigilant state of "freezing" to a more immobile state of "surrender":

John: At first I saw someone walking toward me and it seemed like he began to walk faster so I just focused all my attention on his feet and his hands, made sure I didn't look directly at his face. I thought about moving to the other side of the street but there wasn't time. Then he was just there on top of me. At first I tried to fight him, and get away, but there was nothing I could do. I remember I felt the knife in my chest and then all I know is that my whole body just stopped moving. I think he thought I was dead when he finally left. In some ways, I think I am dead.

This short but direct acknowledgement of John's experience of the physical attack came at a time in the therapy process when he had begun to experience a secure positive attachment within our therapeutic relationship and greater sense of safety to begin to at least imagine discussion of his experience of his body, specifically his experience of "that part of the body is just gone." Equally, if not more, important to the therapy was my own developing professional growth in understanding the "bottom up, not top down" neurobiological functions of the brain in imprinting and processing trauma (Ogden, Minton et al., 2006; Ogden, Pain, & Fisher, 2006; Van der Kolk, 2006; Wylie, 2004). John's ability to cognitively or emotionally process or reassociate with these injured parts of his body (or even be able to experience his torso as part of *his* body instead of *the* body) would only be able to reach a limited point until we first addressed his "here-and-now bodily experience of the traumatic past, rather than its content or narrative" (Ogden, Minton et al., 2006, p. 167) and strengthened his ability to self-observe and remain focused in the present moment versus returning to the familiar response of disconnection or dissociation.

FINDING THE DISSOCIATED BODY FROM THE BOTTOM UP

Van der Kolk studied brain images of patients with posttraumatic stress disorder that actually showed the occurrence of dissociation, the results of which suggested that "when people relive their traumatic experiences, the frontal lobes become impaired and, as a result, they have trouble thinking and speaking. They no longer are capable of communicating to either themselves or to others precisely what's going on" (Wylie, 2004, p. 39). Further neuroimaging studies Van der Kolk collaborated on have also shown that the executive functions of the brain become impaired when traumatized people try to access their trauma. Van der Kolk demonstrated that the imprint of the trauma does not sit in the verbal, understanding, part of the brain, but in much deeper regions—the amygdala, hippocampus, hypothalamus, brain stem—that are only marginally affected by thinking and cognition. These studies showed that people process their trauma from the bottom up—body to mind—not the top down. If trauma is situated in these subcortical areas, then to do effective therapy, therapists need to do things that change the way people regulate these core functions, which probably can not be done by words and language alone. Van der Kolk stressed that much of the work of healing from trauma is "really about rearranging your relationship to your physical self. If you really want to help a traumatized person, you have to work with core physiological states and, then, the mind will start changing" (Wylie, 2004, p. 40).

This understanding and the strong desire to provide a more effective way to more fully relieve John's suffering led me to explore a deeper knowledge of the central role of fixed physiological and sensorimotor patterns in many trauma survivors and possible ways to weave aspects of sensorimotor psychotherapy (Ogden & Minton, 2000; Ogden, Minton et al., 2006; Ogden, Pain et al., 2006) into my foundational response to dissociation through relational trauma psychotherapy (discussed earlier in this article). Ogden, Pain et al. (2006) summarized sensorimotor treatment as follows:

> Sensorimotor treatment focuses on the re-activation of autonomic hyper or hypoarousal and defensive action tendencies as these occur within the therapy hour. In a bottom-up approach, the narrative becomes a vehicle for activating these physiologic responses and movements so that they can be studied and ultimately transformed. The therapist and client have an opportunity to work with the implicit elements of traumatic memories by directing the client's awareness away from the verbal components of memory to the nonverbal residue of the trauma. Somatic bottom-up interventions that address the repetitive, unbidden, physical sensations of hyperarousal and hypoarousal together with movement inhibitions can then be integrated with more traditional top-down interventions that help to transform the narrative of the trauma and facilitate the development of a reorganized somatic sense of self. The sense of self is represented not only in beliefs and emotional responses but also in physical organization, postural habits, and movements of the body. (p. 273)

A much more in-depth understanding of the theory and practice of the sensorimotor approach to psychotherapy is necessary than can be provided within the context of this article. This can be found in the pioneering work by Ogden, Minton et al. (2006), *Trauma and the Body: A Sensorimotor Approach to Psychotherapy*.

The following excerpt from a session with John (about 2 years into therapy) demonstrates the impact of the introduction of this process within our trauma psychotherapy. Specifically, from a sensorimotor perspective this session focused mainly on the recognition and development of "somatic resources for self soothing" (Ogden, Minton et al., 2006, p. 230) to create a safe framework for becoming aware of the body. For John, his relationship with Star had grown to bring a great deal of soothing and an opportunity to build on that physical awareness through an external source.

John: I still can't believe you are letting Star come here. I told her you're a nice person so she should be okay. *[As John took his cat out of the carrier, his body seemed to soften and he gently held her in his lap.]*

Therapist: Well, thanks for that compliment, John. She's beautiful . . . just like you described. And she really seems to like sitting in your lap.

John: Yeah, she's pretty good at always getting my attention.

Therapist: What are you aware of in your body as you notice Star sitting in your lap?

John: I don't really know what you mean, but I know she's getting heavier— I may have to stop giving her so many treats.

Therapist: How do you know she's getting heavier, John—can you feel her weight on your lap?

John: Yeah, I guess so. *[As John answered, his voice trailed off and he seemed to be disconnecting from our conversation while gently rubbing his hand across Star's back.]*

Therapist: John, it seems like something about this is upsetting you. I wonder if we can stop our discussion for just a moment and maybe we could show Star the office.

[I stood up and motioned for John to join me. We walked around the office together, John holding Star, and talked about the many things that Star might experience as toys if we were to let her run free. I handed John different items, encouraging both tactile and verbal connection.]

John: I'm okay to sit back down now, but I don't think we should talk about the lap anymore today.

Although an initial step toward the acknowledgement of John's physical experiencing of self-soothing through his relationship with Star, this session also demonstrates the complexity and crucial importance of pacing the sensorimotor experience and remaining attuned to the client's nonverbal cues much in the same way as in more traditional relational trauma psychotherapy. John and I continued to revisit this session over time with a curiosity and attention to his body's need to physically experience his torso and chest muscles being open and "unguarded" from the danger of being stabbed. Initially, I modeled this physical movement for John and subsequently we practiced the movement together until one session his body sat up with remarkable grace, his chest muscles opened wide, and John described a sense of freedom and relief. He was eventually able to stay grounded and present with the physical sensations in his lap, chest, and hands while petting Star and to utilize his positive internal experience of these sensations for self-soothing. We also continued to build on John's realization that walking and focusing on objects in the room were very useful in reducing the familiar pull toward disconnecting or dissociating from the current moment.

PHYSICALLY CARING FOR THE DISSOCIATED BODY

While we are growing in our understanding of the intrapsychic, the neurobiological and sensorimotor processes connected to dissociation, the experience of "that part of the body is just gone," present an enormous challenge in supporting clients to physically care for their bodies. This dilemma calls upon practitioners of all models of psychotherapy, along with providers of physical medical care, to educate ourselves to recognize the potential "cues" that clients may be disconnected from their physical bodily experience in ways that may have a negative and even progressive impact on the integrity and well-being of their bodies. In other words, we must not actively participate in the intrapsychic function of dissociation that represents *the need not to know*.

In addition to educating ourselves, we must recognize that noticing and naming what is being left out is just as important a premise within relational trauma psychotherapy as noticing and naming interpersonal processes and reenactments that are occurring in the therapy relationship. This implies that therapists take an active role in trying to remain aware of and understand with clients the origins and meanings of clients' self-protective psychological processes, including dissociation. At the same time, therapists must also acknowledge and discuss with clients any actual physical consequences that may have resulted from clients' traumas (Haven & Pearlman, 2004). This concept of noticing and naming what is being left out certainly applies also to other providers who are working with dissociative clients, such as physicians, case managers, bodyworkers, and so on. Unfortunately, many survivors have had traumatic encounters with physical health care providers as adults and may be quite fearful or unwilling to place themselves in an uncertain medical situation. This may necessitate that psychotherapists consider a more active role both in assisting a client to obtain a trauma-informed health care provider and in collaborating with that provider as needed throughout the client's treatment. Additionally, because the psychotherapist is often the only person with whom many clients have disclosed the depth of their traumas, it is a central role of the therapist to provide education and assistance regarding the growing options for collaborative and adjunctive care (such as craniosacral therapy, acupuncture, yoga, massage, integrative medicine, etc.).

As noted earlier, Schnurr and Green's (2004) model depicts the association of traumatic events and poor physical health through psychological, biological, attentional, and behavioral mechanisms and stresses the importance of an integrated approach to care. The authors appropriately stressed that these mechanisms "interact to strain the body's ability to adapt, thereby increasing the likelihood of disease and illness behavior" (p. 268), and they have drawn specific implications for primary care and mental health practitioners, policymakers, and researchers in this arena.

John struggled over several years to effectively care for his physical body. Many things contributed to this struggle: a lack of understanding and education about the specific needs of his body, lack of regular medical check-ups or care, continued smoking, lack of financial resources or adequate medical insurance, lack of exercise, chronic hypoarousal, disconnection from physical pain cues due to dissociation and self-generated analgesia (Haven, 2002; Haven & Pearlman, 2004; Nijenhuis, Vanderlinden et al., 1998; Van der Kolk, 1994), lack of collaborated care among providers, and, yes, a psychotherapist who at some points had to learn along with him about some of the complexities of dissociative experiences, both psychological and physical. Over time, all of these complexities resulted in a medical crisis for John that required an extensive biopsy of his lung—an intrusive procedure on the "part of the body that was just gone." Thankfully, as this possibility became imminent, John, his primary care physician, the specialist who would perform the procedure, and I were able to develop a collaborative process and plan that took into consideration John's particular dissociative coping strategies, his past trauma, and potential emotional and physical triggers and that included my being present with John both before and shortly after the procedure. (This collaboration was possible in large part due to the diligent attention John and I had paid over the years to the complicated process of building a relationship with a primary physician who was compassionate and educated about the impact of trauma.) The following is an excerpt from our discussion about an hour after the procedure while John was still in the recovery room:

John: Well, I guess they cut out whatever they had to and I'm still alive. *[John's facial expression was a slight smile coupled with a sort of grimace that I understood to reflect physical pain.]*

Therapist: You sure are . . . you know, if I'm not mistaken you look like you're both smiling and hurting . . . is that right?

John: *[Looking down at his chest, putting his hand directly over the area of the incision]* They may have taken out part of my chest, but for the first time in a long time, I feel like this part of my body is back . . . I never thought feeling pain could be such a good thing.

CONCLUSION

Empathic engagement and the intimacy of the psychotherapy process with trauma survivors brings a sense of deep respect for the dissociative adaptation that many clients learn as a primary way to tolerate the impact of the suffering and terror they have endured. As therapists we just as deeply understand the ways in which dissociation no longer serves clients well as they strive to heal both psychologically and physically. Not feeling the pain may provide a safe haven from the immediate overwhelming circumstance, but it does not repair the damage or untangle the untold stories held within the body.

My hope in writing this article is to encourage us as psychotherapists to deepen our awareness and overall treatment orientation to include the body as well as the mind and to challenge ourselves to engage with our clients' embodied experiences. It is not enough, and is actually misguided, to focus exclusively on the cognitive and emotional meaning of the experience, the narrative, as the sole entry point to healing. We must understand and act on the reality that past traumatic experiences are indeed imprinted in the deeper regions of the brain that are only marginally affected by thinking and emotion (Van der Kolk, 2006) and are embodied in current physiological states and sensations of hyperarousal and hypoarousal together with movements (or lack of movement) and tissue memories within the body. It is crucial that we assist our clients in giving the body a voice, a visibility; or, as John said, we need to "bring back the part of the body that was gone." The integration of the mind and the body offers the greatest potential for resolving the suffering and long-lasting consequences of trauma and for restoring the innate capacity and desire to move toward health and healing.

NOTE

1. The identity of the client discussed in this article has been disguised by omission and alteration of non-crucial information. I express my sincere gratitude for the client's consent for use within the article of the material that is specific to his or her experience.

REFERENCES

Allen, J. G. (2001). *Traumatic relationships and serious mental disorders.* West Sussex, England: Wiley.

Davies, J. M., & Frawley, M. G. (1994). *Treating the adult survivor of childhood sexual abuse: A psychoanalytic perspective.* New York: Basic Books.

DePrince, A. P., & Freyd, J. J. (2007). Trauma-induced dissociation. In M. J. Friedman, T. M. Keane, & P. A. Resick (Eds.), *Handbook of PTSD: Science and practice* (pp. 135–150). New York: Guilford Press.

Felitti, V. J., Anda, R. F., Nordenberg, D., Williamson, D. F., Spitz, A. M., Edwards, V., et al. (1998). Relationship of childhood abuse and household dysfunction to many of the leading causes of death in adults: The Adverse Childhood Experiences (ACE) Study. *American Journal of Preventive Medicine, 14,* 245–258.

Foa, E. B., Zinbarg, R., & Rothbaum, B. O. (1992). Uncontrollability and unpredictability in post-traumatic stress disorder: An animal model. *Psychological Bulletin, 112,* 218–238.

Goodwin, J. M., & Attias, R. (1999). *Splintered reflections: Images of the body in trauma.* New York: Basic Books.

Haven, T. (2002, November). Physical health and dissociation in relational trauma psychotherapies. In L. A. Pearlman (Chair), *Complex trauma and survivors' bodies.* Symposium conducted at the annual meeting of the International Society for Traumatic Stress Studies, Baltimore, MD.

Haven, T., & Pearlman, L. A. (2004). Minding the body: The intersection of dissociation and physical health in relational trauma psychotherapy. In K. A. Kendall Tackett (Ed.), *Health consequences of abuse in the family: A clinical guide for evidence-based practice* (pp. 215–232). Washington, DC: American Psychological Association.

Levine, P. A. (1997). *Waking the tiger: Healing trauma.* Berkeley, CA: North Atlantic Books.

McCann, I. L., & Pearlman, L. A. (1990). *Psychological trauma and the adult survivor: Theory, therapy, and transformation.* New York: Brunner/Mazel.

Misslin, R. (2003). The defense system of fear: Behavior and neurocircuitry. *Neurophysiologie Clinique, 33*(2), 55–66.

Nijenhuis, E. R. S., Spinhoven, P., Vanderlinden, J., van Dyck, R., & van der Hart, O. (1998). Somatoform dissociative symptoms as related to animal defensive reactions to predatory imminence and injury. *Journal of Abnormal Psychology, 107,* 63–73.

Nijenhuis, E. R. S., Vanderlinden, J., & Spinhoven, P. (1998). Animal defensive reactions as a model for trauma-induced dissociative reactions. *Journal of Traumatic Stress, 11,* 243–260.

Ogden, P., & Minton, K. (2000). Sensorimotor psychotherapy: One method for processing traumatic memory. *Traumatology, 6,* 149–173.

Ogden, P., Minton, K., & Pain, C. (2006). *Trauma and the body: A sensorimotor approach to psychotherapy.* New York: Norton.

Ogden, P., Pain, C., & Fisher, J. (2006). A sensorimotor approach to the treatment of trauma and dissociation. *Psychiatric Clinics of North America, 29,* 263–279.

Pearlman, L. A. (1998). Trauma and the self: A theoretical and clinical perspective. *Journal of Emotional Abuse, 1,* 7–25.

Pearlman, L. A., & Saakvitne, K. W. (1995). *Trauma and the therapist: Countertransference and vicarious traumatization in psychotherapy with incest survivors.* New York: Norton.

Perry, B. D., Pollard, R. A., Blakley, T. L., Baker, W. L., & Vigilante, D. (1995). Childhood trauma, the neurobiology of adaptation, and use-dependent development of the brain: How states become traits. *Infant Mental Health Journal, 16,* 271–289.

Rothschild, B. (2000). *The body remembers: The psychophysiology of trauma and trauma treatment.* New York: Norton.

Saakvitne, K. W., Gamble, S. G., Pearlman, L. A., & Lev, B. T. (2000). *Risking connection: A training curriculum for working with survivors of childhood abuse.* Lutherville, MD: Sidran Press.

Scaer, R. C. (2001). *The body bears the burden: Trauma, dissociation, and disease.* New York: The Haworth Medical Press.

Scaer, R. C. (2005). *The trauma spectrum: Hidden wounds and human resiliency.* New York: Norton.

Scaer, R. C. (2007). *The body bears the burden: Trauma, dissociation, and disease. Second Edition.* New York: The Haworth Medical Press.

Schnurr, P. P., & Green, B. L. (2004). Understanding relationships among trauma, posttraumatic stress disorder, and health outcomes. In P. P. Schnurr & B. L. Green

(Eds.), *Trauma and health: Physical health consequences of exposure to extreme stress* (pp. 247–275). Washington, DC: American Psychological Association.

Van der Kolk, B. (1994). The body keeps the score: Memory and the evolving psychobiology of posttraumatic stress. *Harvard Review of Psychiatry, 1*, 253–265.

Van der Kolk, B. (2006). Clinical implications of neuroscience research in PTSD. *Annals of the New York Academy of Sciences, 1071*(1), 227–293(17).

Wylie, M. S. (2004). The limits of talk: Bessel van der Kolk wants to transform the treatment of trauma. *Psychotherapy Networker, 28*(1), 30–41, 67.

Index